Lynda AOUDIA

Imaging inflammatory breast diseases

Lynda AOUDIA

Imaging inflammatory breast diseases

ScienciaScripts

Imprint

Cover image: www.ingimage.com

This book is a translation from the original published under ISBN 978-620-6-71296-1.

Publisher:
Sciencia Scripts
is a trademark of
Dodo Books Indian Ocean Ltd. and OmniScriptum S.R.L publishing group

120 High Road, East Finchley, London, N2 9ED, United Kingdom
Str. Armeneasca 28/1, office 1, Chisinau MD-2012, Republic of Moldova, Europe
Printed at: see last page
ISBN: 978-620-7-68600-1

IMAGING INFLAMMATORY DISEASES OF THE BREAST

LYNDA AOUDIA

FOREWORD

Inflammatory pathology accounts for around 5% of consultations in breast cancer. The aetiologies are very diverse, corresponding in more than 50% of cases to an infectious origin, most often in the form of simple mastitis, rapidly resolved with medical treatment. In the case of abscesses, ultrasound is the first-line examination, enabling diagnosis and therapeutic intervention, while mammography often shows non-specific signs, and magnetic resonance imaging is only performed in cases where the diagnosis is in doubt. In about 5% of cases, these are inflammatory cancers. These cancers have a poor prognosis and require rapid multidisciplinary management. Clinically, they manifest themselves as inflammatory signs, with oedema, which develop rapidly and are often associated with palpation of a breast or axillary lymph node mass. Mammography reveals suspicious abnormalities. Ultrasound is used to better detect masses and to guide percutaneous biopsy sampling. MRI is used to establish the best extension assessment and post-treatment follow-up. The aim of this book is to present an iconographic review of the various inflammatory breast lesions with radio-histological correlations and to suggest a course of action.

Professor Lynda AOUDIA

TABLE OF CONTENTS

INTRODUCTION

Inflammatory pathology accounts for around 5% of consultations in breast cancer. The aetiologies are very diverse, corresponding in more than 50% of cases to an infectious origin, most often in the form of simple mastitis, rapidly resolved with medical treatment. In the case of abscesses, ultrasound is the first-line examination, enabling the diagnosis and the interventional therapeutic procedures, Mammography shows signs that are usually non-specific, and magnetic resonance imaging (MRI) is only performed in equivocal cases. In about 5% of cases, these are inflammatory cancers. These cancers have a poor prognosis and require rapid multidisciplinary management. Clinically, they manifest themselves as inflammatory signs, with oedema, of rapid onset, frequently associated with palpation of a breast or axillary lymph node mass. Mammography frequently reveals suspicious abnormalities. Ultrasound can help to detect masses within the denser parenchyma and thus guide percutaneous biopsy sampling. Computed tomography (CT) and especially magnetic resonance imaging (MRI) provide the best possible assessment of extension and follow-up under treatment. In other cases, the clinical context and radiological features may help to guide the diagnosis, which is often made using percutaneous sampling.

ANATOMICAL REMINDER

1. BREAST ANATOMY

The breast is a globular organ occupying the anterior-superior part of the thorax. It lies on top of the pectoralis muscle, which holds it in place [1]. It is mainly made up of a mammary gland, supporting connective tissue and adipose tissue, all covered by the skin. The top of the breast is represented by the nipple surrounded by the areola (fig. 1). It is made up of around fifteen main milk ducts, each delimiting a lobe. The mammary ducts open into the nipple at the level of the mammary pores after dilating slightly, forming a lactiferous sinus. Thin fibrous septa separate the lobes, extending into the dermis at the anterior surface of the gland to form Cooper's ligaments, which form Duret's ridges (fig. 1).

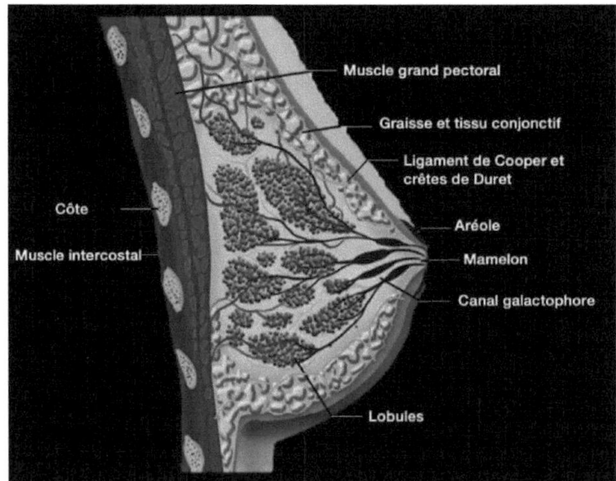

Fig. 1 Anatomical structure of the breast.

2. GALACTOPHORIC TREE

The breast is made up of around fifteen main milk ducts, ending in a nipple pore. These main ducts, after a dilatation known as the lactiferous sinus, branch off into secondary ducts of medium and small calibre up to the Ductulo-Lobular Terminal Unit (DLTU). This UDTL consists of a terminal extra- and intra-lobular galactophore and a lobule made up of around ten alveoli called acini. The UDTL is embedded in a loose connective tissue known as pallaeal tissue. All of this tissue is surrounded by adipose tissue (fig. 2).

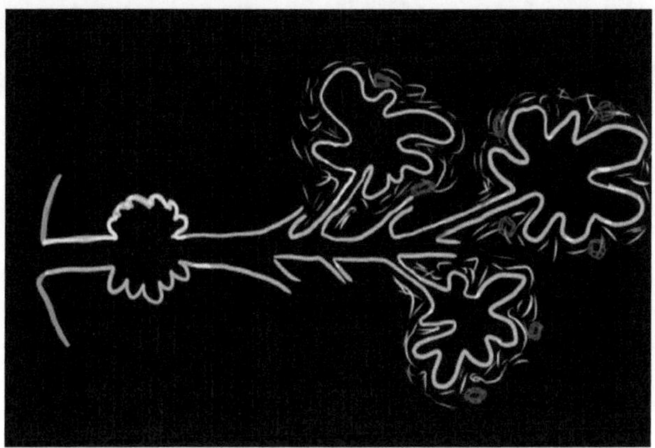

Fig. 2: Diagram of the galactophoric tree.

Histological reminder

The whole of the galactophoric tree is made up of a double layer of cells resting on a basement membrane in direct contact with the blood vessels (fig. 3):

- an inner layer made up of cylindrical epithelial cells responsible for the milk secretory function.
- an outer layer made up of myoepithelial cells responsible for contraction.

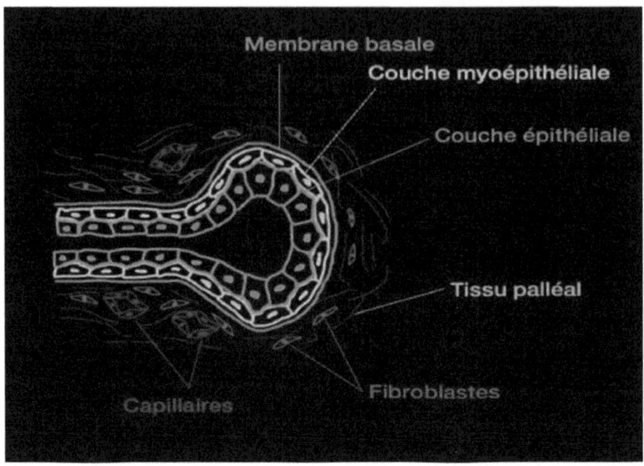

• Fig. 3: Histological diagram of acinar constituents.

IMAGING TECHNIQUES

1. MAMMOGRAPHY

Mammography is the benchmark radiological examination for screening for breast cancer, which is the leading cause of death in women. Mammographic images must be optimised in terms of spatial resolution, contrast and noise. Several technical criteria must be taken into account, in particular, the contrast must be high in order to visualise microcalcifications properly. The radiation spectrum must be broad in order to adapt to the varying densities of the breasts and the minimum radiation dose, especially in young patients.

1.1. Impact

Positioning the breast is a fundamental stage in mammography, and the technique must be beyond reproach. The aim is to radiograph the entire mammary gland, including the deep planes. Positioning is the key to obtaining images of optimum quality, which are essential for interpretation and meet a number of quality criteria [2].

1.1.1. Fundamental impacts

1.1.1.1. Cranio-caudal or frontal incidence

The X-ray beam approaches the breast craniocaudally (fig. 4).

The difficulty with the front view is that the deep mammary planes cannot be seen, so it is important to involve as much posterior mammary tissue as possible. The criteria for successful incidence are (fig. 5):

- The breast is at the centre of the image.

- The gland is well spread out.

- The nipple is at its zenith [3].

- No creases or overlapping.

The pectoralis muscle is visible in almost 30% of cases, and its presence on the image allows optimum depth gain [2].

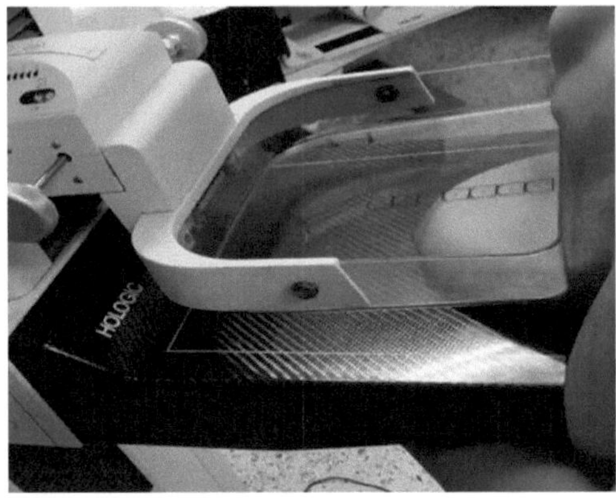

Fig. 4. front view.

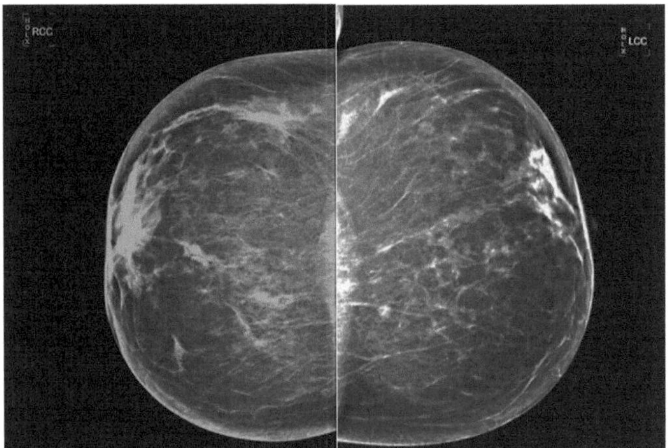

Fig. 5 Quality criteria for the frontal view. Mammographic images. (a) Right side. (b) Left side. Pectoral muscle (1), nipple at zenith (2).

1.1.1.2. 45° external oblique incidence°

This angle allows the breast to be studied in its long axis and a maximum amount of breast tissue to be analysed [4]. The stand is tilted at a strict 45° , to ensure reproducibility (fig. 6). The difficulty with this approach is to compress the pectoral muscle, the breast and the submammary fold evenly.
The criteria for successful incidence are (fig. 7)

- The pectoral muscle is visible up to halfway up the image [5].

- The nipple is at its zenith, opposite the tip of the pectoral muscle [4].

- Presence of the cutaneous fold of the abdominal wall [3].

- The long axis of the breast tends towards the horizontal.

- Presence of the "open" submammary fold, perfectly clear of the abdominal wall [6].

- No creases or overlapping.

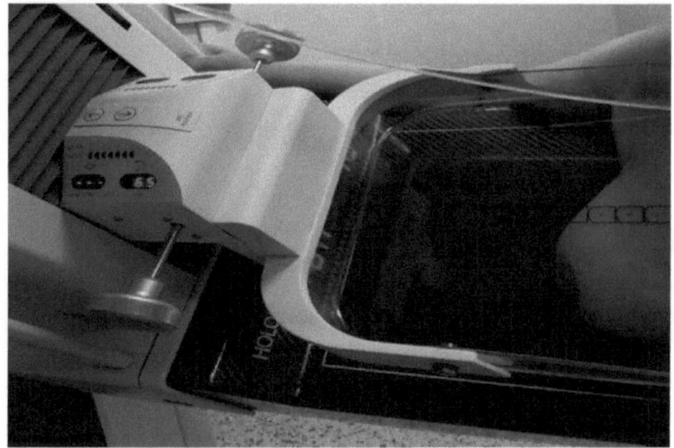

Fig. 6: External oblique incidence.

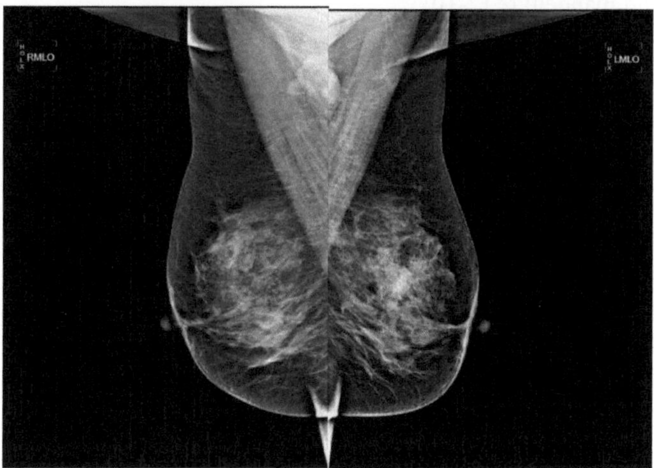

Fig. 7 Quality criteria for external oblique incidence. Mammographic images (a) Right oblique (b) Left oblique. Pectoral muscle (1), skin fold of the abdominal wall (2), open sub mammary fold (3),nipple at the zenith (4).

1.1.2. Additional impacts

They are always carried out in addition to the fundamental impacts.

1.1.2.1. Profile incidence

It is useful for determining the precise location of a lesion. It can also be used to show whether microcalcifications are located in a horizontal position.

1.1.2.2. Centred localized image

It can be used to analyse the contours of a nodule or a stellar image, or to eliminate a constructed image (fig. 8).

1.1.2.3. Enlarged centred image

Microcalcifications visible on standard images can be enlarged for detailed analysis (number, appearance, organisation, etc.) (fig. 9).

1.1.2.4. Other impacts

Axillary extension, Cleopatra incidence, staggered frontal incidence, tangential view, Eklund manoeuvre [7-10].

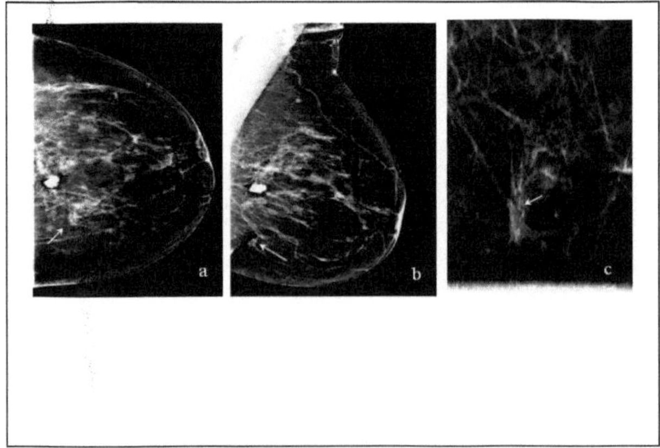

Fig. 8: Centred localized view. (a) Front view. Mass with indistinct contours (arrow). (b) External oblique view. Mass in the sub mammary fold with poorly defined contours (arrow). (c). Centred view located on the mass. Spiculated mass, BIRADS 5 (arrow).

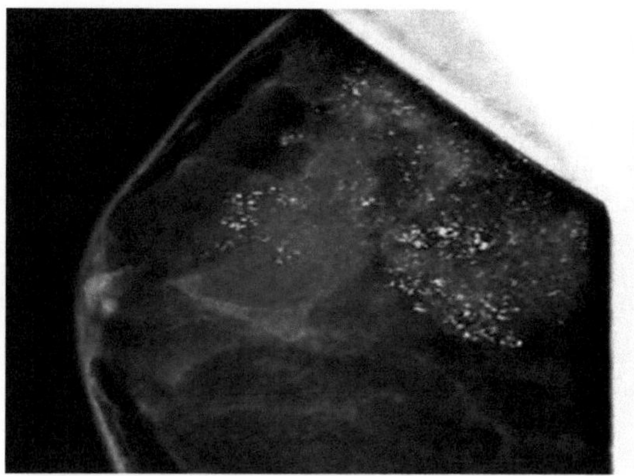

Fig. 9. Enlarged centred view. Magnification of a focus of micro-calcifications.

2. ULTRASOUND

Ultrasound is an accessible, non-irradiating and inexpensive imaging technique. It may be indicated as a complement to mammography, to improve lesion detection, particularly in dense breasts, and to characterise lesions, in particular to differentiate between solid and cystic lesions, and to take samples [11].

Breast ultrasound is performed with a high-frequency probe, usually between 9 and 15 MHz, which provides good contrast and spatial resolution [12]. There are several ultrasound modes.

2.1. Mode B

This is the first technique used when performing breast ultrasound. Ultrasound waves are emitted and collected by the probe, at the same frequency, in a single direction. They are combined to create a 2D image of the breast on a greyscale [13]. This technique allows structures to be differentiated on the basis of the acoustic and mechanical properties of the tissue. This B-mode has a number of weaknesses, including inconsistent optimal resolution and artefacts that can degrade image quality [14] (fig. 10).

2.2. Harmonic mode

It is linked to the non-linear behaviour of breast tissue in relation to ultrasound. As the ultrasound wave propagates through the breast tissue, it undergoes progressive distortion of the shape of the ultrasound pulse, creating harmonic frequencies which are multiples of the emission frequency [15-17]. Once the initial signal has been filtered, the harmonic signal is used to reconstruct the image. This technique improves the contrast of ultrasound images, particularly for cysts with "thick contents" or complicated cysts, which show internal echoes in B mode, whereas in harmonic mode they appear anechoic [18] (fig. 10).

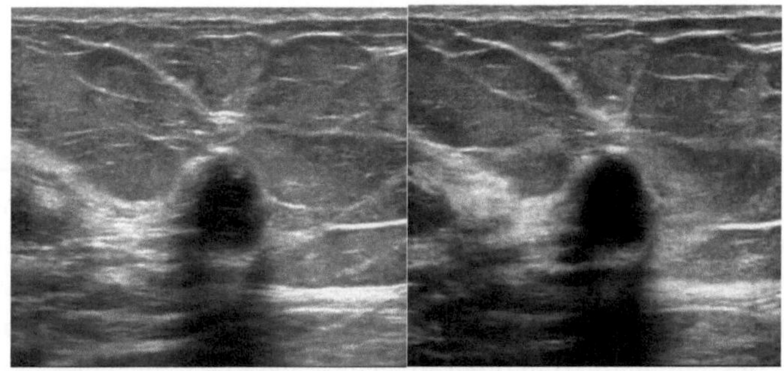

Fig. 10. harmonic mode (a) B-mode ultrasound. hypoechoic mass, (b) Harmonic mode ultrasound. Cystic anechogenic mass with thickened wall. Histology. Histology: remodelled cyst.

2.3. Composite mode (Compound)

There are two types of composite, frequency composite (several different ultrasound emission frequencies are used to reconstruct the final image), and spatial composite (several ultrasound emission angles are used and combined into a single composite image). This technique makes it possible to limit artefacts, improve analysis of lesion contours, better define the internal echostructure of masses and detect small lesions [19] (fig. 11). It also allows better detection of intra-lesional calcifications [20]. On the other hand, posterior ultrasound changes are attenuated [21].

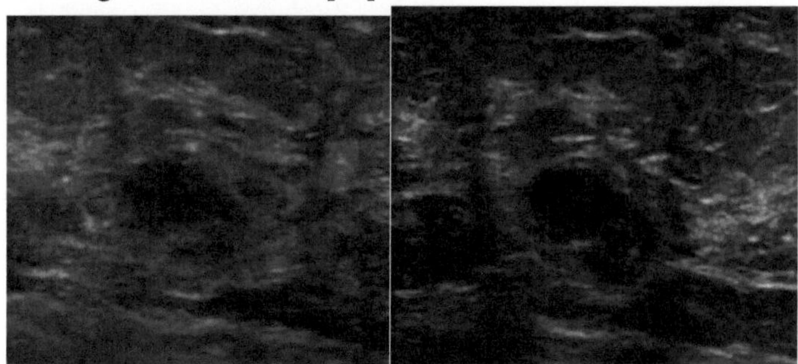

Fig. 11. composite mode. (a) B-mode ultrasound. Hypoechoic mass, at (b) Composite mode ultrasound. Hypoechoic, circumscribed mass. Histology: Adenofibroma.

2.4. Doppler mode

It is used to detect tumour angiogenesis. Malignant lesions are generally more vascularised than benign lesions, with an abnormal, irregular appearance of the vessels. Detection and analysis of the spectrum of these vessels requires a probe of at least 10 MHz and a rigorous ultrasound technique (adjustment of the focal length, reduction of the overall gain, adaptation of the size of the doppler box, filtering to the minimum 10 in order to analyse the low frequencies, no pressure on the breast to avoid obliteration of the small vessels) [22,23]. Energy Doppler has a better sensitivity to slow flows, but is more sensitive to artefacts [24]. Doppler can be used to analyse hypoechoic lesions which pose a "cystic or solid" problem. The presence of vascularisation in an echogenic lesion indicates that the lesion is tissue. On the other hand, the absence of vascularisation does not rule out the presence of a tissue portion [13] (fig. 12).

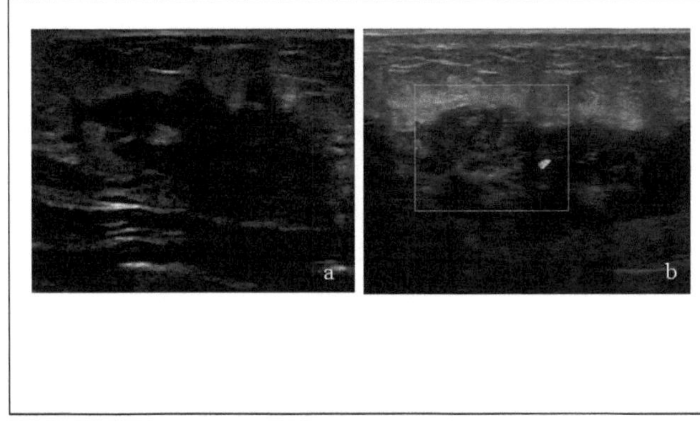

Fig. 12: Doppler mode (a) B-mode ultrasound: hypoechoic mass heterogeneous, with indistinct contours, (b) Doppler mode ultrasound. Intralesional vascularisation.

2.5. Elastography

Elastography is a non-invasive technique used in conjunction with ultrasound to qualitatively, semi-quantitatively or quantitatively assess the deformability of lesions subjected to stress [25, 26]. The image obtained is then translated into an elastogram. This technique was developed with the aim of improving the specificity of B-mode breast ultrasound, by adding to the criteria of echostructure and lesion morphology, the complementary information of compressibility and lesion "hardness" (fig. 13). Breast elastography uses two distinct modes: free-hand elastography and shear-wave elastography.

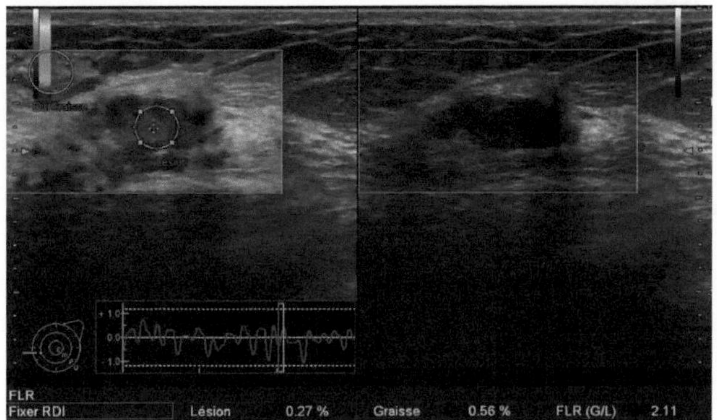

Fig. 13. elastography. Elastography. Calculation of the elasticity ratio in standard deviation.

3. BREAST MRI

3.1. Equipment

3.1.1. Magnetic field

Magnetic field strength affects acquisition time and image quality. The higher the magnetic field strength, the better the image resolution and the shorter the sequences. Most teams work with magnetic fields of 1.5 tesla (T).

3.1.2. Antennas

Breast MRI should be performed using dedicated breast antennas that follow the shape of the breasts (fig. 14). The use of parallel imaging improves the performance of these antennas, increasing the area covered, signal uniformity, and temporal and spatial resolution [27]. The breasts must be well positioned in the antenna, with the nipple at the zenith, integrating the entire breast into the antenna and avoiding folds (fig. 15).

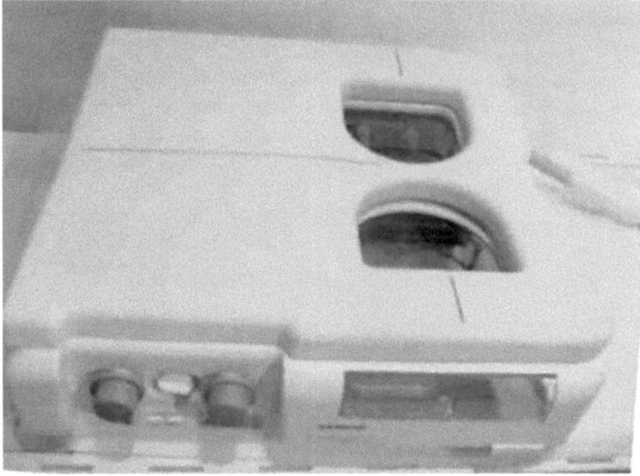

Fig. 14. Antenna breast.

The breast should not be compressed too much. Compression serves to support the breasts to prevent their movement in the antenna. Excessive compression of the breast can falsely reduce the size of lesions and thus change the TNM classification [28]. Compression can also reduce the amplitude of enhancement and modify the enhancement curve (fig. 16).

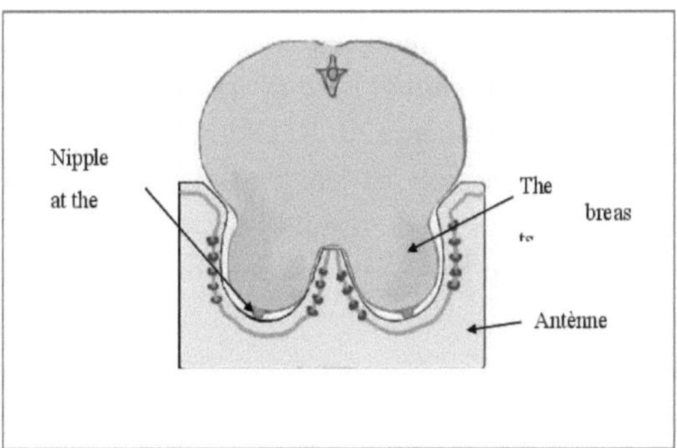

Fig. 15. Position of the breasts in the anterior.

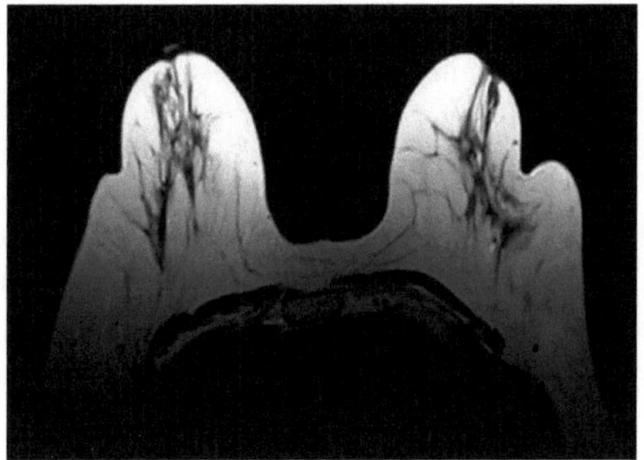

Fig. 16. Compression defect. T2-weighted sequence.

3.2. Time of the examination

The timing of the examination is essential for a better interpretation of breast MRI. The second part of the cycle should be avoided, when physiological glandular enhancement is most marked. It is minimal in the 2nd week of the menstrual cycle in patients who are genitally active. Outside this period, there may be diffuse non-specific contrast, but also focal contrast, which may lead to misinterpretation (fig. 17). Glandular enhancement is increased by hormone replacement therapy in postmenopausal women, by up to 50 % of women have non-specific enhancements. A 3-month stop in the event of an uninterpretable examination in post-menopausal women.For post-operative MRI, a minimum delay of one month should be observed to limit enhancement secondary to inflammatory phenomena; the optimal time for performing breast MRI is at least six months after the end of treatment [29- 31].Percutaneous microbiopsies do not generally affect the interpretation of contrast-enhanced MRI. However, the topography, date of biopsies and results, if available, should always be mentioned. Oral contraception also has no impact on the use of breast MRI.

3.3. Settling the patient

A venous access with a long tube is put in place. The patient is then placed in the procubitus position, with her arms over her head as comfortably as possible, to ensure the immobility required for the examination. The breasts placed in the antenna must be well supported; if necessary, a foam pad can be used to prevent the small breasts from moving in the antenna.

3.4. Injection of contrast medium

Breast MRI highlights intratumoral neoangiogenesis by injecting a contrast agent, enabling lesions to be detected [32]. The contrast agent used is gadolinium chelate. The dose injected is 0.1 mmol/kg body weight. The injection rate should be 2 to 3 ml per second. The injection of the contrast product is followed by an injection of 20 ml of physiological saline at the same rate to avoid stagnation of the contrast product in the tubing.

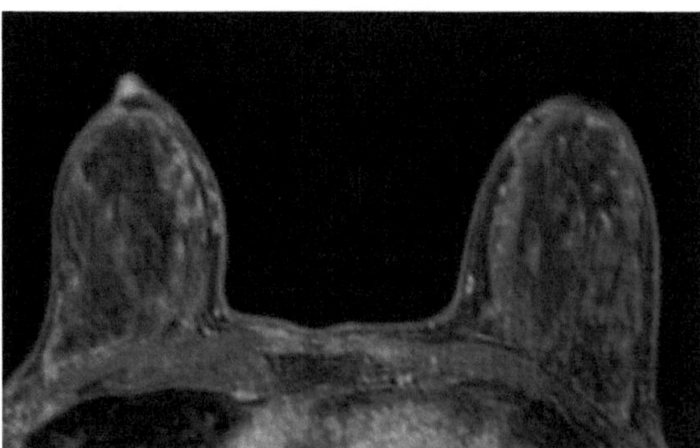

Fig. 17. Enhancement glandular enhancement. Subtracted sequence injected

3.5. Breast MRI protocols

3.5.1. Acquisition plan

The fields of view must be wide enough to analyse both breasts, both nipple-areolar plates (NAPs), the axillary hollows and the chest wall [32, 33]. Acquisition in the axial plane is the most frequently used. This acquisition plane makes it possible to carry out dynamic sequences of the breasts in 1 minute. The advantages of the axial plane are that the entirety of both breasts can be analysed comparatively, which makes it easier to detect abnormal contrast, and also allows analysis of the PAM, the axillary fossae and the chest wall [33]. Cardiorespiratory artefacts degrade the quality of acquisitions. Phase encoding from right to left instead of anteroposterior reduces these artefacts. Acquisition in the sagittal plane makes it possible to reduce the field of view. This improves image resolution and the quality of fat suppression techniques [32]. Finally, sagittal acquisition also allows better analysis of physiological glandular enhancement, which facilitates anatomical study. Nevertheless, the study of both breasts with the axillary hollows requires a large number of slices, which prolongs the examination time [33].Coronal acquisition reduces cardiac artefacts. However, this plane is often degraded by respiratory and flow artefacts. This acquisition plane also requires a lot of slices to be able to analyse the entire breast from the chest wall to the PAM [33].

3.5.2. Cutting thickness

The slice thickness must be thin, less than or equal to 3 mm, with a pixel and voxel size of less than 1 mm. This will enable us to carry out multiplanar reconstructions.

3.5.3. Breast MRI sequences

3.5.3.1. Morphological sequences

In the past, non-injected T2- and T1-weighted sequences in breast MRI were not considered very useful because of their poor diagnostic value. Since then, many authors have demonstrated the value of using morphological sequences.

T2-weighted sequences can be used to detect cystic lesions, the presence of which indicates benign enhancement, whether annular enhancement in inflammatory cysts or non-mass enhancement in fibrocystic mastopathy (figs. 18 and 19).T2-weighted sequences with fat saturation are very useful in the case of nipple discharge, making it possible to create indirect MRI galactography images and also improve the detection of small cancers (fig. 20). T1-weighted sequences without fat saturation are useful for detecting the presence of a fatty component in a lesion, which is an important factor in favour of benignity (fig. 21). These sequences are also useful for confirming the correct position of metal markers in the biopsy site [34] (fig. 22).

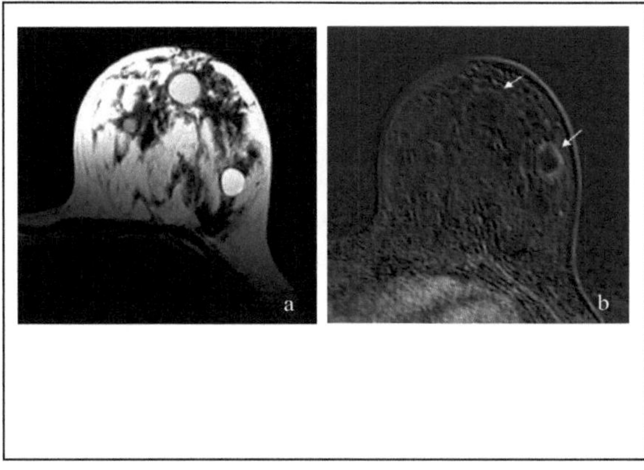

Fig. 18. Inflammatory cysts. (a) T2 sequence, (b) injected subtraction. Round lesions with T2 hypersignal and annular enhancement after injection of contrast medium (arrows).

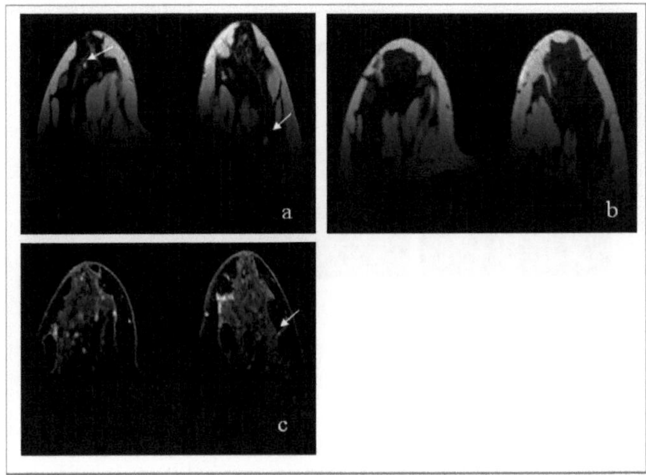

Fig. 19. fibrocystic mastopathy.
(a) T2 sequence, (b) T1 sequence, (c) T1 Fat Sat sequence after injection of contrast medium. Multiple microcysts in T2 hypersignal, hyposignal T1 with presence of multiple enhancements not mass

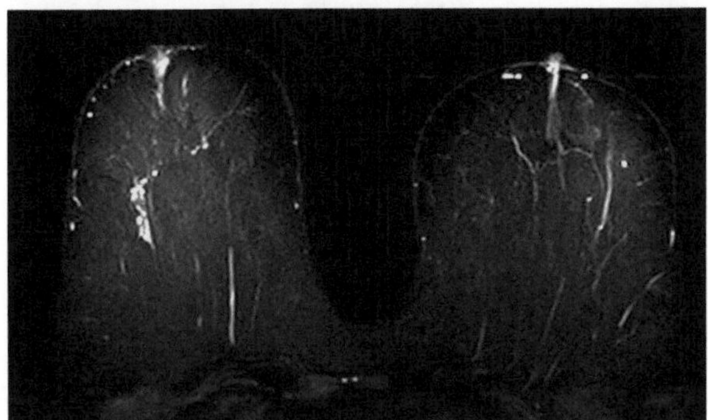

Fig. 20. Ductal ectasia. Intracanal hypersignal on T2 sequences with fat suppression (arrows).

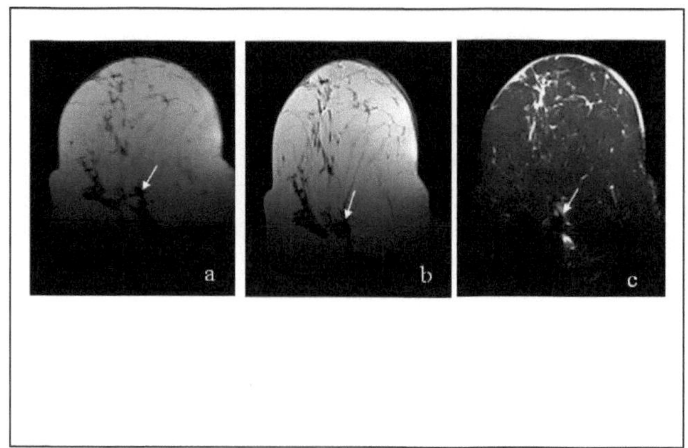

Fig. 21 Cytosteatonecrosis: (a) T1 sequence, (b) T2 sequence, (c) T2 Fat Sat sequence. Lesion in T1 hypersignal, T2 hypersignal, in hyposignal on the T2 sequence with fat suppression (arrows).

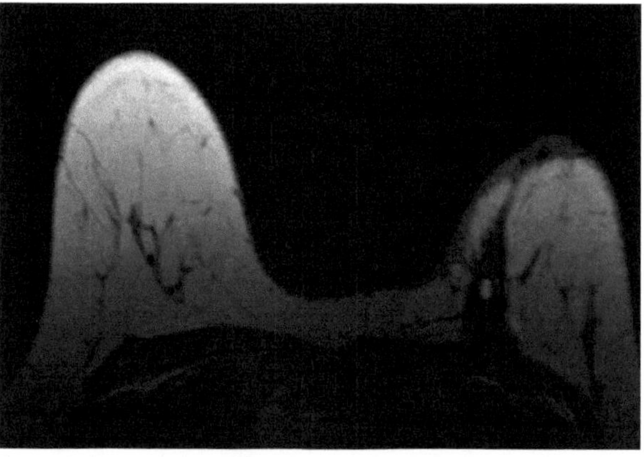

Fig. 22. Position of the metal marker in the ground on the T1 sequence (arrow).

3.5.3.2. Dynamic sequences

Dynamic analysis makes it possible to distinguish suspicious abnormal angiogenesis from the various enhancement kinetics. T1 gradient echo sequences after injection of gadolinium chelate (fig. 23).2D or 3D acquisition? Compared with 2D sequences, 3D sequences give finer slices with a better signal-to-noise ratio [32]. However, since 3D acquisition is performed without fat suppression, it is advisable to use 2D sequences to reduce the phase encoding artefacts that extend in all three directions in 3D sequences, masking the contours and making it difficult to detect these artefacts on subtraction sequences. The 3D sequence enables the lesion to be analysed in volume (measurement in the 3 planes, distance from the nipple-areolar plate and the deep pectoral plane) (fig.24).

3.5.3.3. Complementary sequences

- **Broadcast**

The principle of diffusion imaging is to quantify the movement of water molecules in tissues. The objectives of diffusion sequences are to optimise the detection of small lesions and improve the characterisation of benign and malignant lesions. Diffusion MRI can also be used to assess the response to neoadjuvant chemotherapy. An increase of more than 10% in ADC coefficients at the end of the first cycle of chemotherapy indicates a decrease in cell density, and is therefore predictive of response to treatment [35, 36].

- **Magnetic resonance spectroscopy**

Spectroscopy is a molecular imaging technique. Its principle is to detect an abnormal choline peak in malignant tumours (resonance at 3.2 ppm) [37]. Bartella et al. reported that adding spectroscopy to the standard protocol improved the PPV of biopsies from 35% to 82% ($p<0.01$) and enabled biopsy to be avoided in 57% of lesions [38]. In addition, numerous studies have shown that this sequence can demonstrate an early response (at 24 h) to neoadjuvant chemotherapy [64].

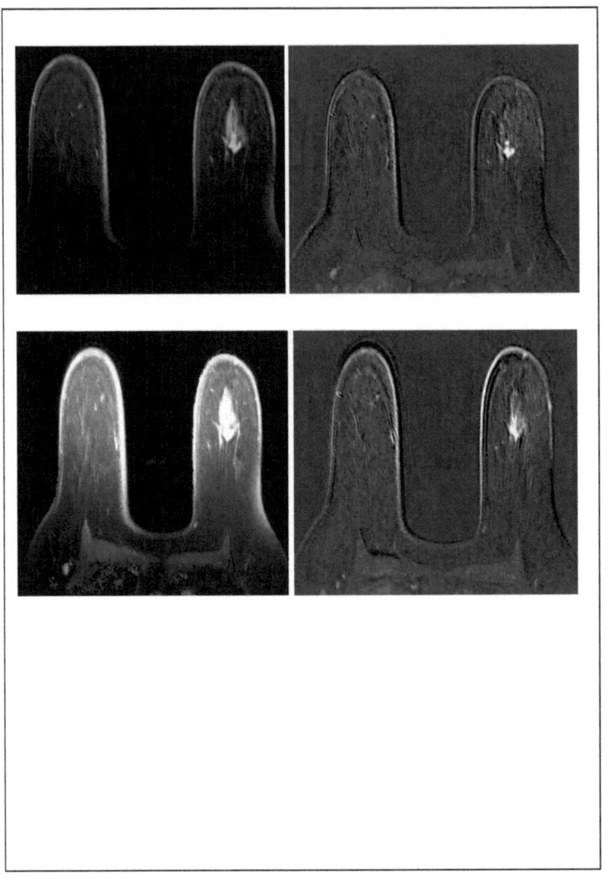

Fig. 23. Enhancement analysis of a malignant tumour of the left breast. Dynamic analysis makes it possible to distinguish the tumour from the rest of the fibroglandular parenchyma thanks to acquisition before the second minute in three-dimensional (3D) T1 weighting (a) and injected 3D T1 with subtraction (b). At six minutes, it is difficult to differentiate the cancer from the breast parenchyma on the injected 3D T1 (c) and injected 3D T1 with subtraction (d) sequences.

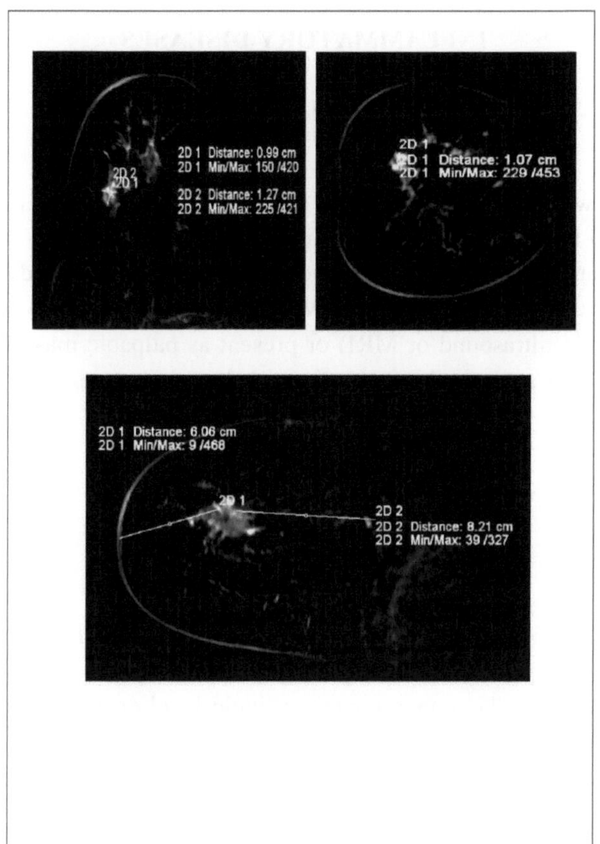

Fig. 24. Injected 3D T1-weighted sequence with subtraction. The volume of the lesion is analysed (measurement in the 3 planes (a + b), the distance of the lesion from the nipple-areolar plate and the deep pectoral plane (c).

INFLAMMATORY DISEASES

1. INFLAMMATORY CYST

One third of women aged between 30 and 50 have breast cysts [40]. They are very common between the ages of 30 and 40, and may diminish with the onset of the menopause. They are linked to the dilatation of a lobule or duct, forming a cyst. They are most often discovered during screening examinations (mammography, ultrasound or MRI) or present as palpable masses. On clinical examination, it is not possible to distinguish between a cyst and a solid mass [41, 42].

1.1. Imaging

Ultrasound is the best test for making the diagnosis [40]. Inflammatory cysts or complicated cysts present all the aspects of simple cysts, but with contents that are finely echogenic. They may contain a liquid level or more or less abundant internal echoes which move when the patient changes position and which correspond to debris, or they may contain thick echogenic liquid imitating a solid lesion [43] (figs. 25, 26, 27). Finally, it may be a thick-walled cavity (fig. 28). This cyst is often under tension and painful when the catheter is passed. Puncture allows the cavity to be evacuated, a cytological diagnosis of benignity to be made and healing to be accelerated. On colour echodoppler, significant hypervascularisation can be seen around the cyst (figs. 26, 28). On elastography, the cyst often shows a blue-green-red artefact, reflecting the fluid nature of the cystic contents (fig. 27). Several studies have demonstrated that any lesion showing a blue-green-red artefact on elastography is a cystic lesion [44, 45]. The authors have proposed that the presence of this artefact can differentiate a cystic lesion from a solid lesion [44, 45]. On MRI, the inflammatory cyst appears as a T1 hypposignal, T2 hypersignal lesion with an enhanced wall after injection of contrast medium (figs. 29, 30).

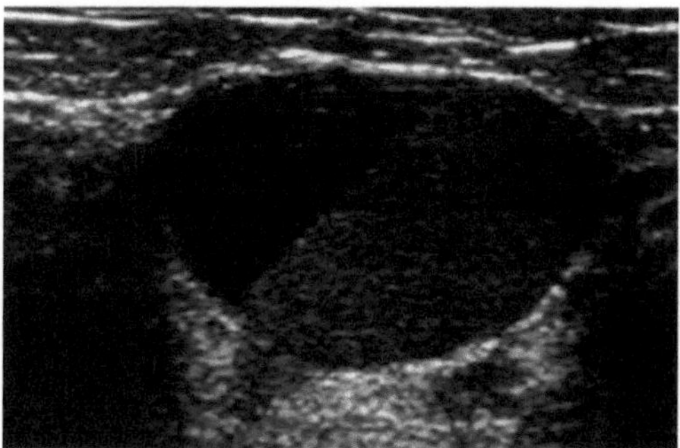

Fig. 25. Inflammatory cyst. Ultrasound mode B. An ovoid mass with an imperceptible wall, showing a liquid/liquid level, hypoechoic in the depressed region (arrow) with posterior enhancement (asterisk) [46].

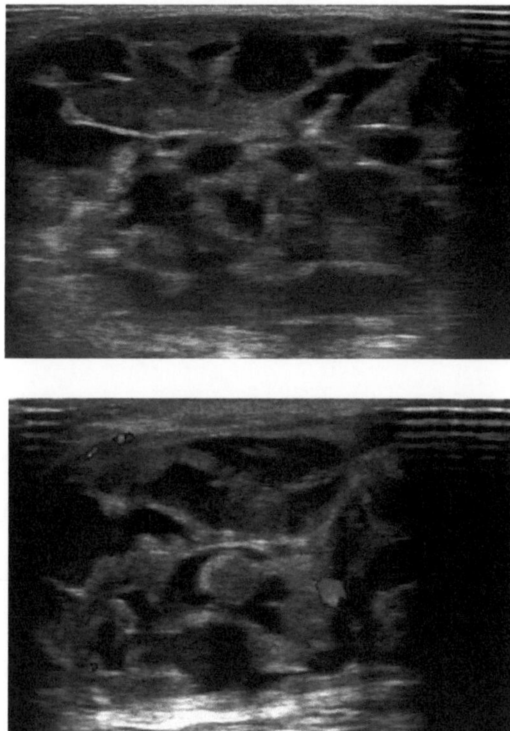

Fig. 26. Inflammatory cyst. (a) B-mode ultrasound. Cyst with thick septa (arrows). (b) Doppler ultrasound. Mass with peripheral vascularisation.

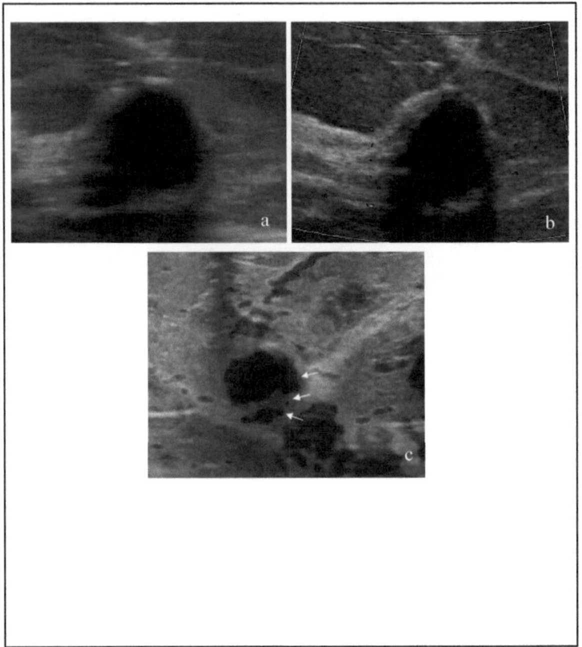

Fig. 27. Inflammatory cyst. (a) B-mode ultrasound. Round mass with circumscribed contours, long axis perpendicular to the skin, hypoechoic, abrupt interface, no posterior acoustic effect, classified BIRADS 4a. (b) Colour Doppler. Non-vascularised lesion in Doppler mode. (c) Elastography. Blue-green-red artefact at the site of the lesion.

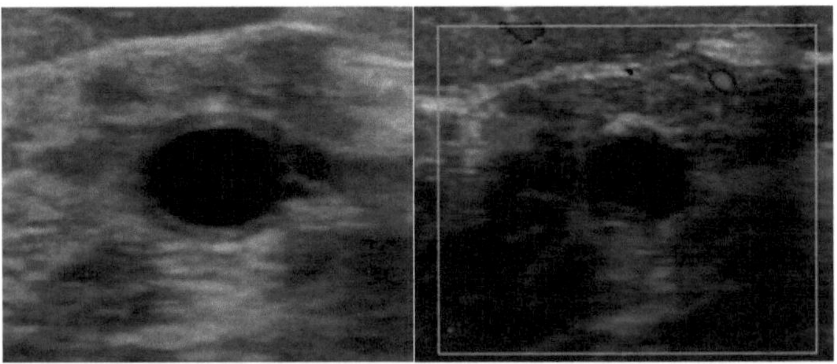

Fig. 28. Inflammatory cyst. (a) B-mode ultrasound. Round cystic lesion, with circumscribed contours, delimited by a thick echogenic wall (arrow). (b) Colour Doppler. Non-vascularised mass.

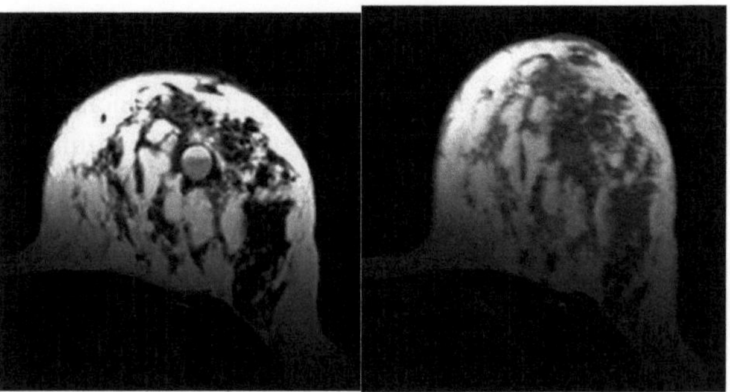

Fig. 29. Inflammatory cysts. MRI (a) T2 sequence, (b) T1 sequence. Cystic lesion with an oval shape and circumscribed contours, presenting a liquid level. Different signals on T2 and T1 sequences (arrows).

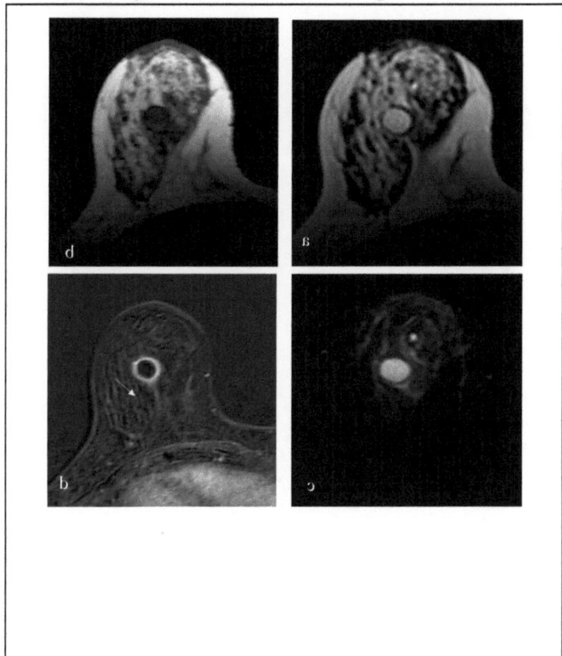

Fig. 30. Inflammatory cyst. (a) T1-weighted sequence. (b) T2-weighted sequence. (c) T2 Fat Sat-weighted sequence. (d) Injected subtraction sequence. Round lesion with circumscribed contours, hypersignal T2 and T2 Fat Sat, hypposignal T1, thickened wall, hypposignal T1 and T2.
ring enhancement after injection of contrast (arrow).

1.2. What to do

If the inflammatory cyst is under tension and painful, puncture can be used to evacuate the lesion, make a cytological diagnosis of benignity and speed up healing.

2. INFECTION OF A GALACTOCELE

Galactoceles are the most frequent benign pathology secondary to breastfeeding. They most often occur after breastfeeding has stopped or during breastfeeding and during the third trimester of pregnancy. They are cystic ductal dilatations, filled with milk.

2.1. Imaging

Their ultrasound appearance may be anechoic, with thin walls and posterior enhancement, or echogenic and heterogeneous, with a fat-liquid level (fig. 31). They may become infected, and the clinical examination will show inflammatory phenomena, with a heterogeneous appearance on ultrasound, with thickened walls and vascularisation on Doppler. Sometimes, solid necrotic tissue can be seen within the pus [47] (fig. 32). Elastography usually shows a soft lesion (fig. 32).

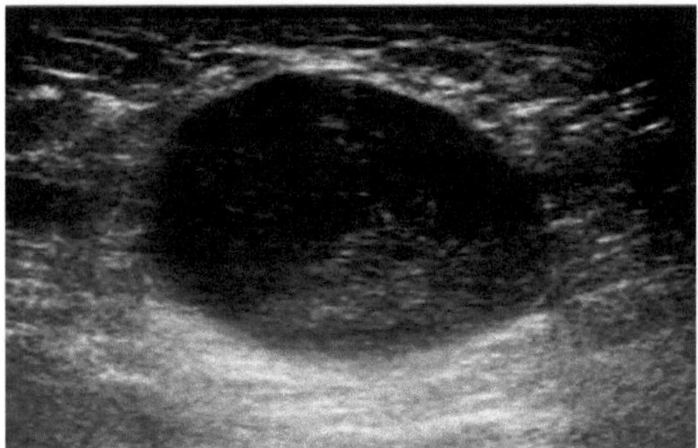

Fig. 31. Superinfected galactocele. B-mode ultrasound. Cystic lesion, anechogenic, with thick hypoechoic content with internal echoes and a liquid-liquid level within it, with abrupt interface with enhancement. posterior acoustic (asterisk).

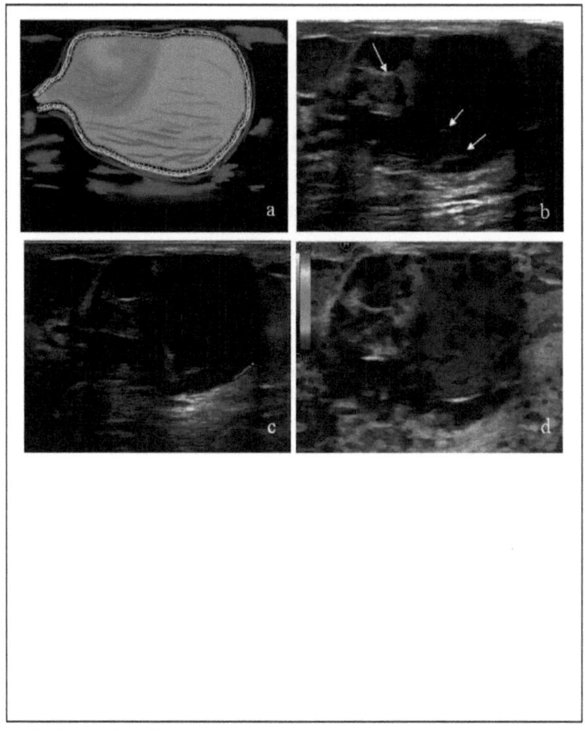

Fig. 32. Superinfected galactocele. (a) Diagram. Cystic ductal dilatation with superinfected fluid content and debris within (asterisk). (b) B-mode ultrasound. Cystic lesion, anechoic, with thick hypoechoic content and internal echoes that shift with changes in position (arrows), with abrupt interface and posterior acoustic enhancement. (c) Colour Doppler. The hypoechoic portion is not vascularised. (d) Elastography. Soft score lesion of elasticity 2.

2.2. What to do

Percutaneous or surgical drainage accompanied by appropriate antibiotic therapy [47, 48].

3. INFLAMMATION OF A LACTATING ADENOMA

Lactating adenoma is a benign lesion that occurs during pregnancy or post partum. Its true nature is controversial. Some authors suggest that it corresponds to a variant of fibroadenoma, tubular adenoma or lobular hyperplasia with changes associated with pregnancy. Histologically, it is a well circumscribed lobular proliferation consisting of a compact aggregate of lobules and secretory hyperplasia. Characteristically, it regresses spontaneously. It may undergo necrotic and inflammatory changes.

3.1. Imaging

On mammography, a lactating adenoma generally appears as a fibroadenoma-like, oval mass with its long axis parallel to the skin and regular contours. On ultrasound, the lesion is heterogeneous (fig. 33). In some cases, there are fatty areas within the lesion, suggestive of the diagnosis, which are radiolucent on mammography and echogenic on ultrasound. These areas correspond to milk fat secreted as a result of hyperplasia. In some cases, it may present more equivocal aspects, particularly in cases of necrosis [48-51].

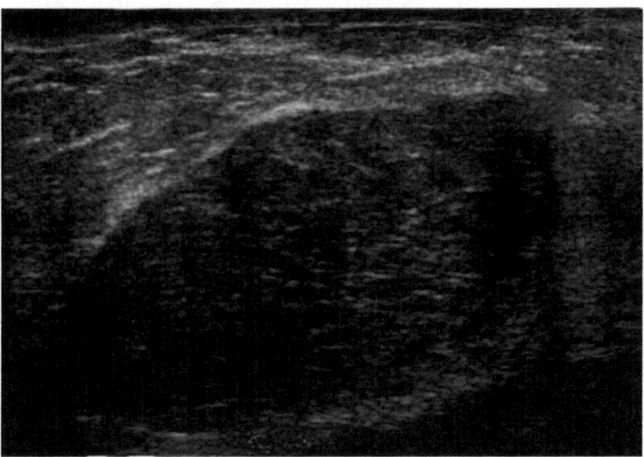

Fig. 33. Inflammation of the lactating adenoma. Ultrasound mode B. Heterogeneous hypoechoic mass with discreetly indistinct contours in a pregnant woman.

4. ABSCESS

Mammary abscesses are purulent collections formed in the breast [52]. A distinction is made between lactating or puerperal abscesses, which occur during breastfeeding, and non-lactating or non-puerperal abscesses. The causes are generally bacterial infections, tuberculosis and, exceptionally, mycotic or parasitic infections [53, 54]. Clinically, abscesses are most often marked by local oedema, erythema and pain, but suppurative forms may occur from the outset [52, 55]. Palpation usually reveals a poorly defined mass.

4.1. Imaging

Diagnosis of an abscess is essentially ultrasonographic, demonstrating a hypoechoic, rounded lesion with more or less irregular contours, usually of heterogeneous echostructure, with a thickened wall [56]. Abscesses may fistulate into the skin, visible as tubular anechoic structures in contact with the abscess (fig. 34). Ultrasound can also be used to puncture or drain the abscess [57, 58]. Elastography confirms the benign nature of the lesion, which is generally flexible. On MRI, the abscess appears as a thick-walled mass with a T1 hypposignal and T2 hypersignal, which is enhanced after injection of contrast medium (Fig. 35).

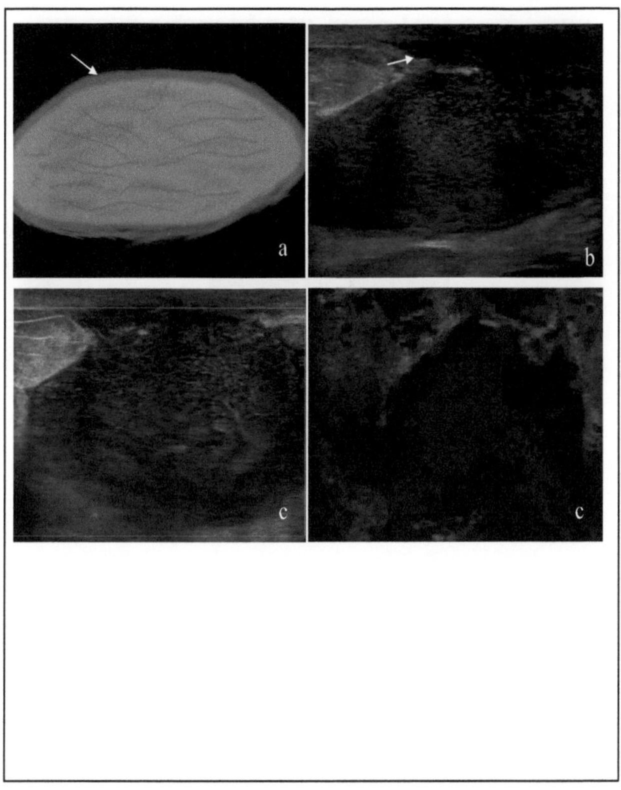

Fig. 34. Abscess (a) Diagram. Purulent collection with a thick wall (arrow). (b) B-mode ultrasound. Hypoechoic mass, with circumscribed contours and fistulised to the skin (arrow), with abrupt interface and posterior acoustic enhancement. (c) Colour Doppler. Non-vascularised mass. (d) Elastography. Mass flexible.

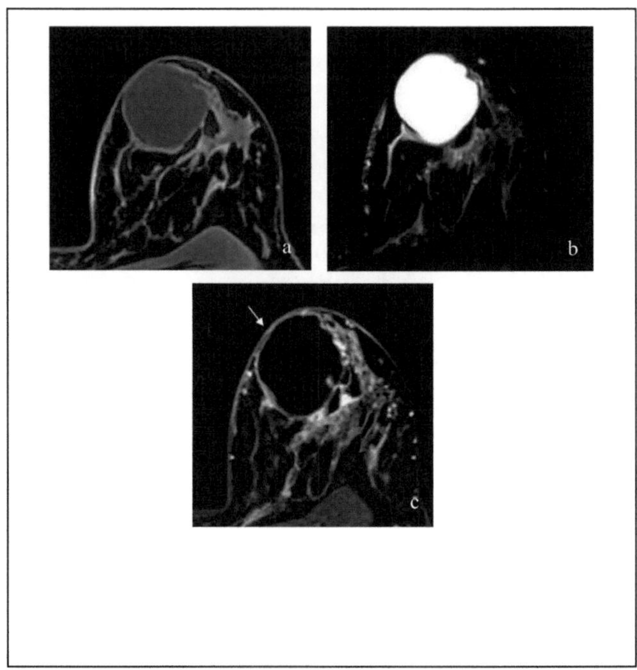

Fig. 35. Abscess. MRI: (a) T1 sequence, (b) T2 STIR sequence, (c) injected subtraction sequence. Round cystic lesion with T1 hyposignal, T2 hypersignal, surrounded by a thick wall and enhanced after injection of contrast medium. (arrow).

4.2. What to do

A monitoring ultrasound should be initiated under treatment treatment (antibiotic and anti-inflammatory therapy) [59]. Following the episode, a full conventional check-up should be carried out to eliminate any residual treatment. If a lesion persists, samples should be taken to rule out a progressive process [42].

5. CYTOSTEATONECROSIS

A benign, non-infectious inflammatory lesion of traumatic origin, secondary to surgery, radiotherapy or trauma [40-42]. It generally occurs in post-menopausal women [40-42]. Clinically, it appears as a palpable, poorly defined mass, sometimes adherent to the skin, round and superficial, mimicking a cancer [40-42].Histologically, the fat initially undergoes necrosis, becoming hard, followed by an inflammatory infiltrate rich in macrophages and giant cells, and finally fibrosis, the retractile nature of which gives it a worrying appearance. Sometimes the central area liquefies, causing cavitation (oily cyst).

5.1. Imaging

Mammography shows a clear, rounded breast, sometimes with a stellate mass which may contain a few amorphous calcifications. Ultrasound shows a low echogenic image with no variation in the posterior acoustic bundle in the early stages (fig. 36). As fibrosis sets in, the lesion becomes more echogenic, often heterogeneous with posterior attenuation, mimicking a malignant lesion [40, 42] (fig. 36). In this case, elastography often reveals a soft lesion (Fig. 37). Cytosteonecrosis on MRI is manifested by a T1, T2 hypersignal lesion with a drop in signal on T2 Fat Sat sequences (fig. 38).

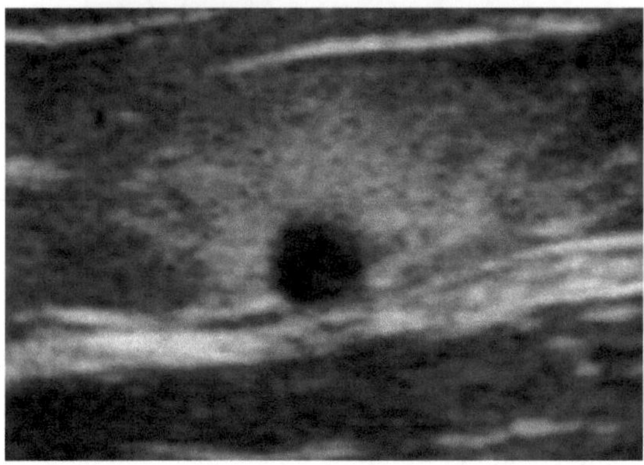

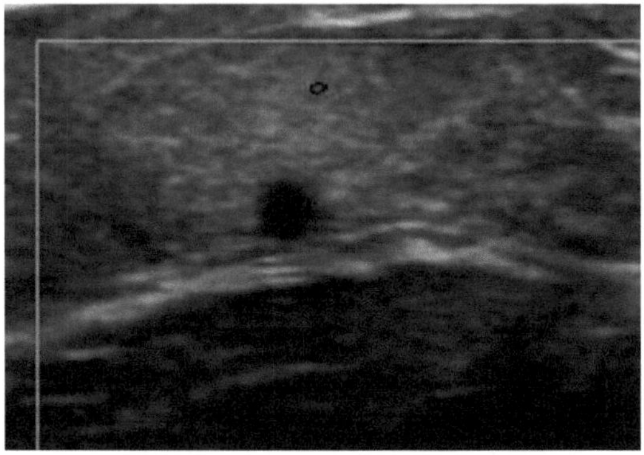

Fig. 36. Cytosteatonecrosis. Early stage (a) Ultrasound mode B. Ultrasound. Echogenic cyst surrounded by hyperechoic peripheral fat (arrow). (b). Colour Doppler. Non-vascularised mass.

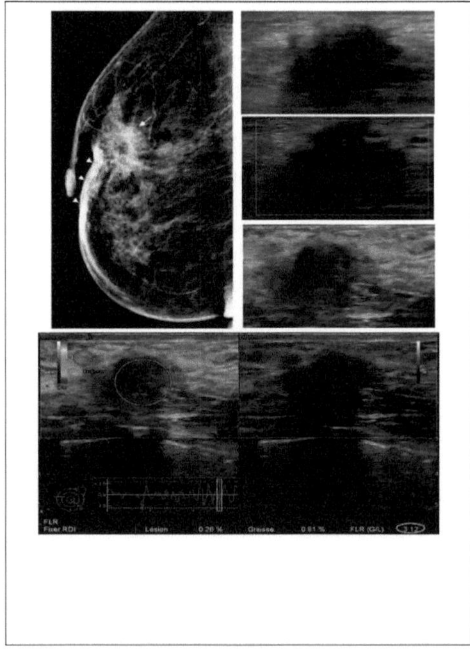

Fig. 37. Cytosteatonecrosis. Late stage (a) Mammogram. Hyperdense mass with irregular shape and contours (arrow) associated with thickening and skin retraction (arrowheads). (b) B-mode ultrasound. Highly hypoechoic mass with irregular contours, attenuating, imitating a malignant mass. (c) Colour Doppler. Non-vascularised mass. (d+e) Elastography. Mass of intermediate hardness, elasticity score 3 and elasticity ratio 3.12.

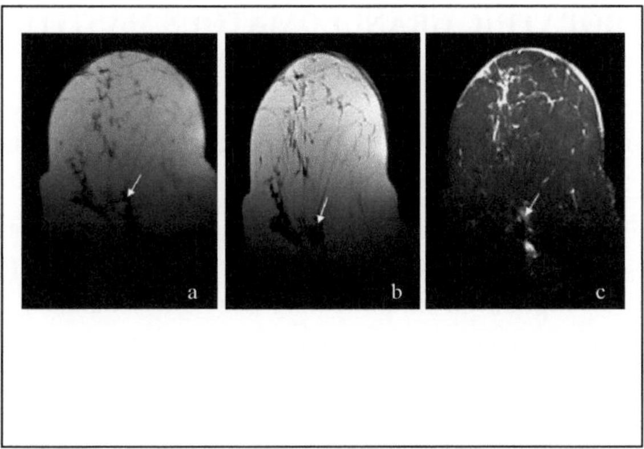

Fig. 38. Cytosteatonecrosis: (a) T1 sequence, (b) T2 sequence, (c) T2 Fat Sat sequence. Lesion in T1 hypersignal, T2 hypersignal, in hyposignal on the T2 sequence with fat suppression (arrows).

5.2. What to do

In the absence of radio-clinical discordance, surgical abstention may be proposed in cases of cytosteatonecrosis. No recommendation can be made regarding the monitoring of a cytosteatonecrosis lesion.

6. IDIOPATHIC GRANULOMATOUS MASTITIS

Idiopathic granulomatous mastitis is a rare chronic inflammatory lesion, accounting for 1% of inflammatory breast diseases [60]. It most often occurs in young women, during periods of genital activity [61]. Little is known about the aetiopathogenesis of idiopathic granulomatous mastitis. Several hypotheses have been put forward to explain an inflammatory reaction secondary to hormonal, metabolic, traumatic or mechanical factors [62]. An auto-immune process has also been suggested [63]. The most frequent mode of revelation is the appearance of a clinically suspicious mass, associated with adenopathy.Its inflammatory form is rarer and can develop into repeated aseptic abscesses, fistulating in the skin. Histologically, these are epithelioid granulomas without caseous necrosis, associated with a polymorphic inflammatory infiltrate consisting of plasma cells, lymphocytes and neutrophils [64].

6.1. Imaging

Mammography in the inflammation stage shows an overall increase in breast density associated with thickening of the skin covering. Sometimes a homogeneous, well-limited mass can be seen, sometimes with spiculated contours or disorganisation of the trabeculae. Mammographic findings in granulomatous mastitis are non-specific. It is most often a poorly defined asymmetry of density, without microcalcifications or architectural distortion (fig. 39).Interpretation is more difficult in young women, whose breasts are dense, especially if the condition is bilateral, On B-mode ultrasound, granulomatous mastitis usually appears as a heterogeneous hypoechoic mass (figs. 39, 40). Multifocal abscess and adenopathy may be seen. Imaging findings are often suspicious of malignancy [65] (fig. 40). MRI may be of secondary interest in eliminating an underlying tumour process, which may be an infiltrating lobular carcinoma. However, the examination may be rendered difficult if there is persistent residual inflammation. In this case, radial biopsies may be useful.

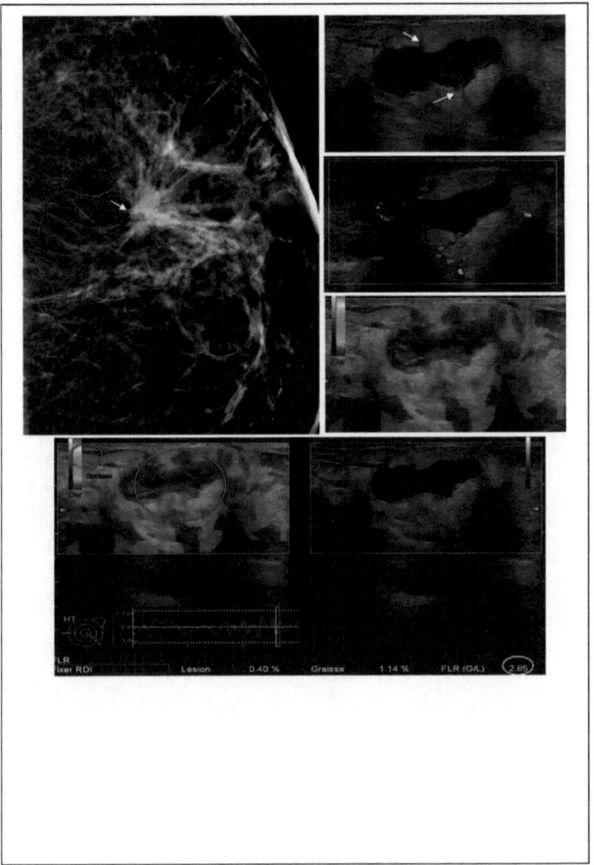

Fig. 39. Idiopathic granulomatous mastitis (a) Mammogram. Hyperdense, irregularly shaped mass with spiculated contours (arrow). (b) B-mode ultrasound. Hypoechoic mass, with angular contours (arrows) and a large hyperechoic peripheral halo (asterisk), classified as BIRADS 5. (c) Colour Doppler. Mass with peripheral vascularisation, at the level of the hyperechoic halo. (d+e) Elastography. Mass showing a blue-green-red artefact, suggestive of fluid content, surrounded by a halo of intermediate hardness. The elasticity ratio is estimated at 2.85.

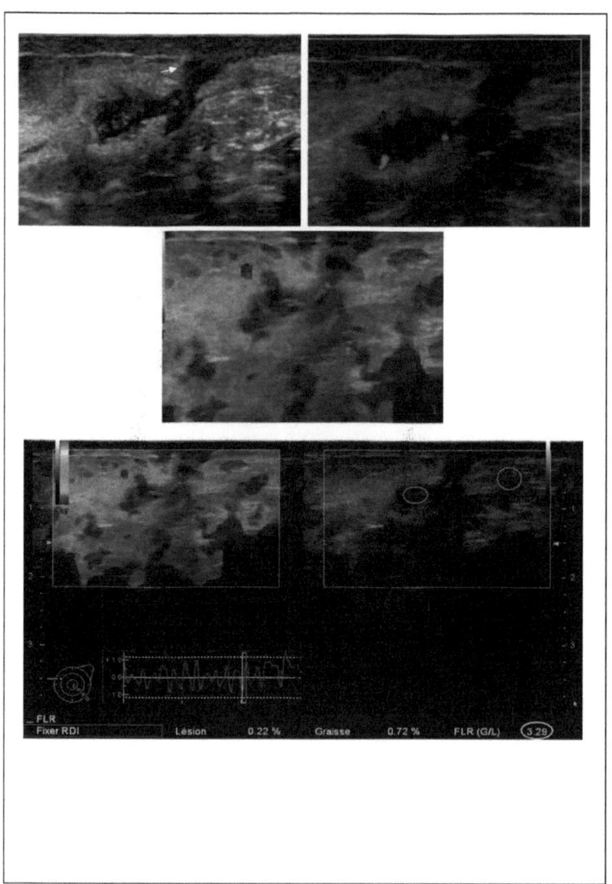

Fig. 40. Idiopathic granulomatous mastitis: (a) B-mode ultrasound. Hypoechoic mass, irregular in shape, with spiculated contours and fistulae in the skin (arrow), a hyperechoic peripheral halo (asterisk), classified as BIRADS 5. (b) Colour Doppler. Mass with peripheral vascularisation. (c+d) Elastography. Soft to intermediate hardness mass, elasticity score 2 and estimated elasticity ratio 3.29.

6.2. What to do

Treatment is exclusively medical. There is no indication for surgical treatment. On the contrary, surgical intervention could increase the risk of non-healing and recurrence [66].Treatment consists of non-steroidal anti-inflammatory drugs until healing. Some authors have obtained good results with corticosteroid therapy [67]. There is no indication for antibiotic treatment unless superinfection is proven.In the case of a collected abscess, the microbial pus can be evacuated using a large needle or a small scalpel incision. Methotrexate is still of real interest in cases where corticosteroid therapy has failed [68].

7. LIPOGRANULOMA

Lipogranuloma is a subcutaneous lesion, clinically manifested as a poorly limited nodule or plaque, yellowish in colour, adherent to the skin and mobile deep down, and may be complicated by ulceration or suppuration. Lipogranuloma is seen in obese women, frequently following haematoma or trauma, sometimes even minor. Cold may be a contributing factor. Histological examination shows necrosis of fat cells in the hypodermis, associated with a macrophagic reaction of the foreign body type, with a clear tendency towards sclerosis [69].

7.1. Imaging

On ultrasound, it presents as a hyperechoic, heterogeneous, well circumscribed mass (fig. 41). The mass is generally soft on elastography.

7.2. What to do

No recommendations can be made regarding monitoring.

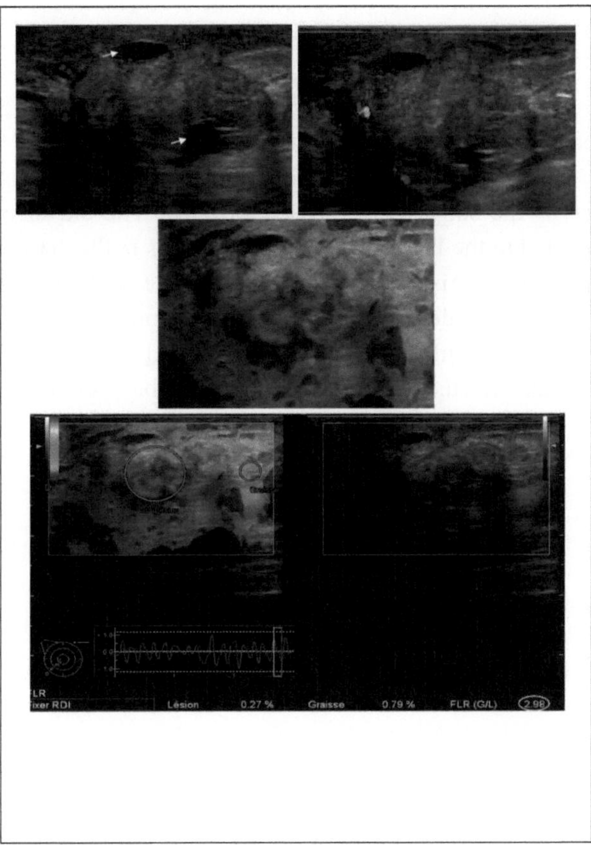

Fig. 41. Lipogranuloma. (a) B-mode ultrasound. Oval, hyperechoic mass with macrolobulated contours, containing cystic areas (arrow), associated with thickening of the skin (asterisk). (b) Colour Doppler. Vascularised mass in Doppler mode. (c+d) Elastography. Soft mass, elasticity score 2 and estimated elasticity ratio 2.98.

8. EPIDERMAL CYST

Epidermal cysts are a frequent benign skin lesion, preferentially located on the scalp and forehead. Mammary localization is rare [70].The histogenesis of epidermal cysts is the subject of much controversy. The old theory suggested that skin trauma led to the inclusion of epidermal cells in the dermis. These cells continue to grow, giving rise to cysts, hence the name epidermal inclusion cyst. In the breast, cases of epidermal cysts have been reported after breast reduction and microbiopsy. Currently, this theory is refuted by certain authors and epidermal cysts and related lesions are thought to be pilosebaceous or sweat adnexal lesions [71]. Histologically, the epidermal cyst is a cystic cavity bordered by a regular squamous lining, filled with blades of keratin, sebum and dead cells [71].

8.1. Imaging

À The ultrasound scan shows a superficial, rounded or oval, circumscribed mass. It often contains abundant echoes which might suggest a solid lesion were it not for the context and superficial location (fig. 42).

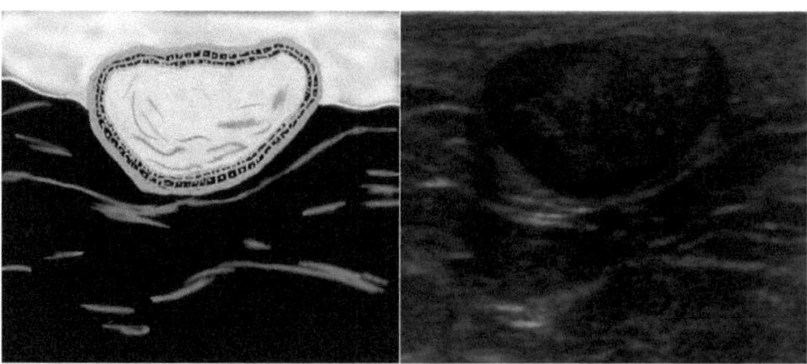

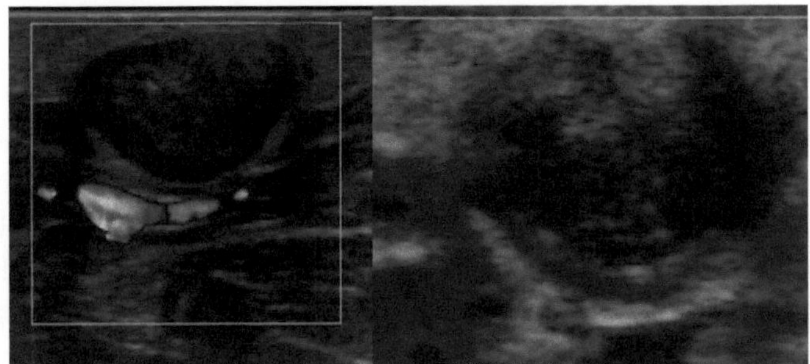

Fig. 42. Epidermal cyst (a) Diagram. Subcutaneous cyst containing sheets of keratin, sebum and dead cells (asterisk), bordered by squamous cells (black arrow) and surrounded by a capsule (red arrow). (b) B-mode ultrasound. Subcutaneous hypoechoic mass, oval in shape, with circumscribed contours, classified as BIRADS 3. (c) Colour Doppler. Non-vascularised mass on Doppler (d) Elastography. Intermediate hardness mass, elasticity score 3.

8.2. What to do

The rupture of an epidermal inclusion cyst or a sebaceous cyst can result in intense inflammation and abscess formation. Treatment is essentially surgical, based on monobloc resection of the A lesion. The histological study is mandatory because of the possibility of association or malignant transformation [71].

9. INFLAMMATORY BREAST CANCER

Inflammatory cancers are a rare form, accounting for 1-5% of breast cancers. Clinically, they are characterised by the rapid appearance of an inflamed, red, warm, oedematous and painful breast, which should be distinguished from locally advanced cancers with secondary inflammatory signs [72]. They occur most often between the ages of 45 and 54. Associations have been described with overweight and smoking.Histological diagnosis is based on the demonstration of tumour cell emboli in the dermal lymphatic vessels. All histological types are possible, with non-specific infiltrating carcinomas predominating. Tumours are usually poorly differentiated, high grade, with negative hormone receptors, strong HER2 overexpression and higher levels of EGF receptors [72]. Clinically, inflammatory skin changes are observed, progressing rapidly over a few weeks: thickened, oedematous skin, infiltrated like orange peel skin, oedema predominating in the lower regions and, in the area of the areola-mammary plate, erythema localised to the tumour or extending to the whole breast, or even to the contralateral breast, which may take on a purplish or brownish appearance, with an increase in local heat. The breast is often painful, with possible retraction of the nipple-areolar plate. Venous circulation may be increased, with dilated vessels. In around 60% of cases, a mass is palpable, and in over 50% of cases, an axillary or supra-clavicular lymph node is palpable. Generally, these manifestations occur without fever [72].

9.1. Imaging

On mammography, there are aspecific changes associated with inflammation, such as skin thickening, stromal infiltration, architectural disorganisation or a diffuse increase in density, and more characteristic tumour changes with mass syndromes, malignant-looking microcalcifications or adenopathies [73] (fig. 43).On ultrasound, there are non-specific skin and subcutaneous changes, such as skin thickening, dilation of lymphatics and veins, interstitial oedema and hyperechoic subcutaneous fat; there are also parenchymal changes, such as focal attenuation without mass, reflecting stromal infiltration [73] (fig. 44). Above all, it is possible to identify masses that are often irregular, heterogeneous and vascularised, which are easier to detect than in mammography, particularly in the case of dense breasts, allowing samples to be taken for histological purposes [73-78] (fig. 45). On MRI, non-specific inflammatory changes are seen, with thickening of the skin that takes contrast after injection, a diffuse T2 hypersignal associated with oedema, an increase in breast volume, hypervascularisation and diffuse contrast enhancement. Focal contrast is often found, in up to 100% of cases in some studies, in the form of a mass and non-mass enhancement [75, 76, 78-83] (fig. 46). MRI provides a better assessment of tumour extension and therapeutic response, as well as diagnosing any contralateral lesions.

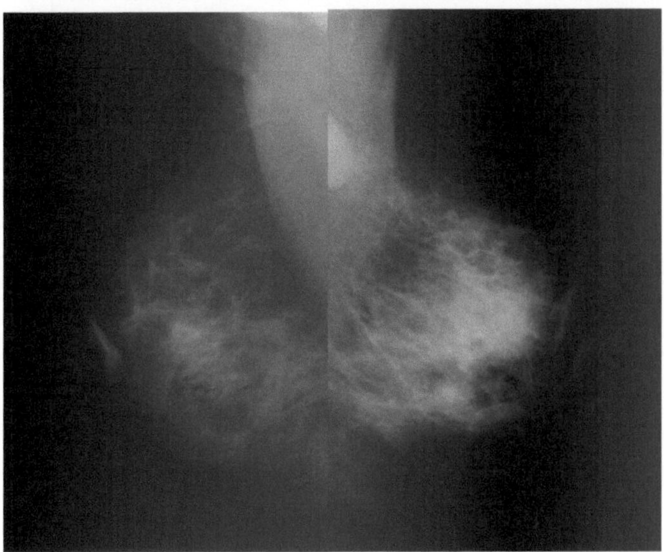

Fig. 43. Inflammatory cancer. (a+b) Oblique mammography Mass of the breast left breast, poorly limited associated à a infiltrate stromal infiltrate, skin thickening and axillary adenopathy (arrows) [84].

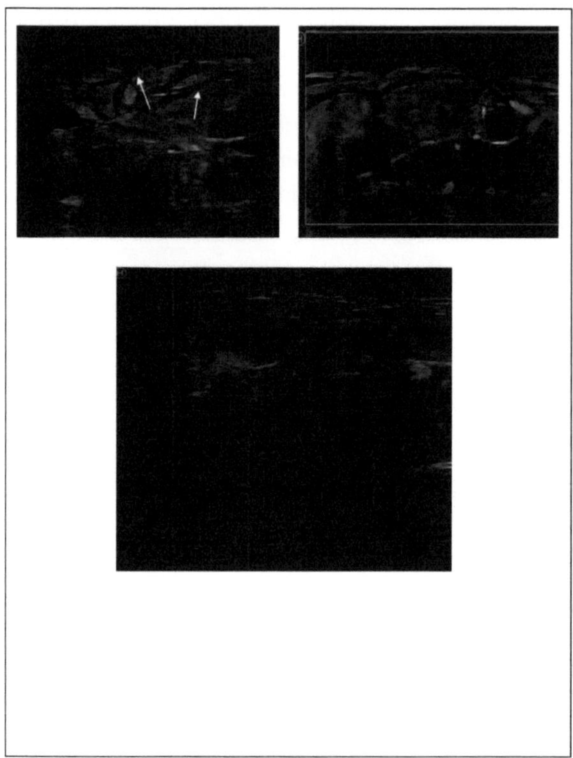

Fig. 44. Inflammatory cancer. (a) Ultrasonography. Thickening of the skin with hyperechoic appearance of the subcutaneous fat and dilation of the lymphatic channels (arrows). (b) Colour Doppler. Hypervascularisation of the subcutaneous fat. (c) Ultrasound. Focal attenuation without mass, reflecting stromal infiltration.

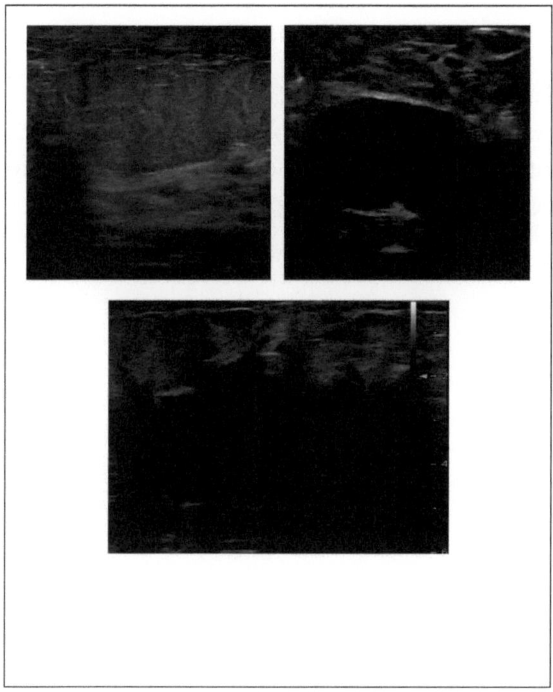

Fig. 45. Inflammatory cancer. (a) Thickening of the skin with hyperechoic subcutaneous fat and discrete dilation of the lymphatic channels. (b) Axillary adenopathy. (c) Attenuating malignant mass, irregular in shape, with irregular contours.

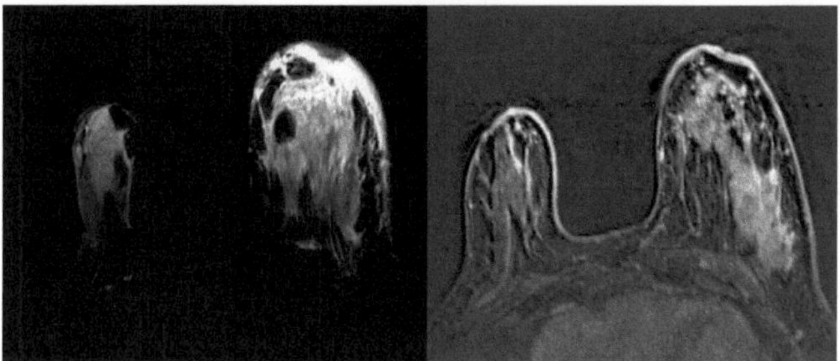

Fig. 46. Inflammatory cancer. (a) Fat Sat T2-weighted sequence. (b) Injected subtraction sequence. Left unilateral oedema with hypersignal T2 Fat Sat on the injected sequences, showing a mass suspicious of malignancy of irregular shape and contours, with heterogeneous enhancement (arrow) associated with thickening of the skin and vascular dilatation under the skin.

9.2. Progression and course of action

The prognosis is poor, with early metastatic progression in 30 per cent of cases. of cases. Five-year survival is 30-50%, obtained with rapid multidisciplinary management, with neoadjuvant chemotherapy followed by locoregional treatment varying according to the therapeutic response [72].

REFERENCES

1. Couturaud B, Fitoussi A. Anatomy / surgery of breast cancer. Conservative treatment, oncoplasty. Surgical techniques in gynaecology. Elsevier Masson; 2011 ; 4-7.

2. Baur A, Bahrs SD, Speck S, Wietek BM, Kremer B, Vogel U, et al. Breast MRI of pure ductal carcinoma in situ: sensitivity of diagnosis and influence of lesion characteristics. Eur J Radiol 2013;82:1731-7.

3. Hammersleya JA, Partridgeb SC, Blitzera GC, Deitcha S, Rahbarb H. Management of high-risk breast lesions found on mammogram or ultrasound: the value of contrast-enhanced MRI to exclude malignancy. Clinical Imaging 49; 2018; 174-
180. https://doi.org/10.1016/j.clinimag.2018.03.011

4. Andolina VF, Lill√© SL, Willison KM, Mammographic Imaging. A practical guide. 2 nd ed. Lippincott Williams and Wilkins; 2001.

5. Austin C. R and Short R. V. Hormonal Control of Reproduction. 2nd edition of Reproduction in Mammals, Vol.3. Cambridge: Cambridge University Press. 1984.

6. Faulconer LS, Parham CA, Connor DM, Kuzmiak C, et al. Effect of breast compression on lesion characteristic visibility with diffraction-enhanced imaging. Acad Radiol 2010; 17 (4) : 433-40. Epub 2009 Dec 29.

7. Kinzelin S. Positioning, the √©tape cl√© of the mammography examination. Imagerie du sein Elsevier Masson, 2012; 2: 19-27.

8. Mancuso S, Ottolenghi G. The oblique projection in the radiologic Study of the breast. Minerva Ginecol 1989; 41 (7): 325-8.

9. Konguth PJ, Rimer BK, Conaway MR, et al. Impact of patient-controlled compression on the mammography experience. Radiology 1993; 186 (1): 99-102.

10. Muntz EP, Logan WW, Focal spot size. And scatter supression in magnification mammography. AJR Am J Roentgenol 1979; 133 (3): 453-9.

11. Corsetti V, Houssami N, Ferrari A, Ghirardi M, Bellarosa S, Angelini O, et al. Breast screening with ultrasound in women with mammography-negative

dense breasts: evidence on incremental cancer detection and false positives, and associated cost. Eur J Cancer. 2008 Mar;44(4):539-44.

12. Athanasiou A, Tardivon A, Ollivier L, Thibault F, El Khoury C, Neuenschwander S. How to optimize breast ultrasound. Eur J Radiol. 2009 Jan;69(1):6-13.

13. Weinstein SP, Conant EF, Sehgal C. Technical advances in breast ultrasound imaging. Semin Ultrasound CT MR. 2006 Aug;27(4):273-83.

14. Sehgal CM, Weinstein SP, Arger PH, Conant EF. A review of breast ultrasound. J Mammary Gland Biol Neoplasia. 2006 Apr;11(2):113-23.

15. Amersham Health. Encyclopaedia of Medical Imaging. http://eu.aershamhealth/com/medcyclopaedia/

16. Clevert DA, Jung EM, Jungius KP, Ertan K, Kubale R. Value of tissue harmonic imaging (THI) and contrast harmonic imaging (CHI) in detection and characterisation of breast tumours. Eur Radiol 2007 ; 17 : 1-10.

17. Rosen EL, Soo MS. Tissue harmonic imaging sonography of breast lesions: improved margin analysis, conspicuity, and image quality compared to conventional ultrasound. Clin Imaging. 2001 Nov-Dec;25(6):379-84.

18. Athanasiou A, Balleyguier C. Nouveaut√© techniques en √©chographie mammaire. Imagerie de la Femme. 2007;17(4):247-54.

19. Huber S, Wagner M, Medl M, Czembirek H. Real-time spatial compound imaging in breast ultrasound. Ultrasound Med Biol 2002; 28: 155-63.

20. Cha JH, Moon WK, Cho N, Chung SY, Park SH, Park JM, et al. Differentiation of benign from malignant solid breast masses: conventional US versus compound imaging. Radiology 2005;237:841-6.

21. Balu-Maestro C. Bases de l'àö¬©chographie mammaire. Imager ie du sein. Paris: Elsevier-Masson; 2012. p. 101-17.

22. Dickinson RJ, Hill CR. Measurement of soft tissue motion using correlation between A-scans.Ultrasound Med Biol 1982;8(3):263-71.

23. Krouskop TA, Dougherty DR, Vinson FS. A pulsed Doppler ultrasonic system for making noninvasive measurements of the mechanical properties of soft tissue. J Rehabil Res Dev 1987;24(2):1-8.

24. Ophir J, C√©pedes I, Ponnekanti H, Yazdi Y, Li X. Elastography: a quantitative method for imaging the elasticity of biological tissues. Ultrason

Imaging 1991;13(2):111-34.

25. Youk JH, Gweon HM, Son EJ. Shear-wave elastography in breast ultrasonography: the state of the art. Ultrasonography. 2017 Oct;36(4):300-309. doi: 10.14366/usg.17024.

26. Tristant H, Benmussa M, Bokobsa J, Elbaz P. Variation of the normal breast: mammographic and √©chographic appearance. Encycl M√©d Chir 1994; 810-G-15.

27. Sardanelli F, Boetes C, Borisch B, Decker T, Federico M, Gilbert FJ, et al. Magnetic resonance imaging of the breast: recommendations from the EUSOMA working group. Eur J Cancer. 2010 May;46(8):1296-316.

28. El Khouli RH, Macura KJ, Kamel IR, Bluemke DA, Jacobs MA. The effects of applying breast compression in dynamic contrast material-enhanced MR imaging. Radiology 2014;272:79-90.

29. Wilkinson J, Appleton CM, Margenthaler JA. Utility of breast MRI for evaluation of residual disease following excisional biopsy. J Surg Res 2011;170:233-9.

30. Lee JM, Orel SG, Czerniecki BJ, Solin LJ, Schnall MD. MRI before reexcision surgery in patients with breast cancer. AJR Am J Roentgenol 2004;182:473-80.

31. Orel SG, Reynolds C, Schnall MD, Solin LJ, Fraker DL, Sullivan DC. Breast carcinoma:MRimaging before re-excisional biopsy. Radiology 1997;205:429-36.

32. Kuhl C. The current status of breast MR imaging. Part I. Choice of technique, image interpretation, diagnostic accuracy, and transfer to clinical practice. Radiology. 2007 Aug;244(2):356-78.

33. Mann RM,Kuhl CK, Kinkel K, Boetes C. Breast MRI: guidelines from the European Society of Breast Imaging. Eur Radiol 2008;18:1307-18.

34. Szumowski J, Coshow W, Li F, Coombs B, Quinn SF. Double-echo three-point- Dixon method for fat suppression MRI. Magn Reson Med 1995;34(1):120-4.

35. Sharma U, Danishad KK, Seenu V, Jagannathan NR. Longitudinal study of the assessment by MRI and diffusion-weighted imaging of tumor response in patients with locally advanced breast cancer undergoing neoadjuvant chemotherapy. NMR Biomed 2009;22:104-13.

36. Iacconi C, Giannelli M, Marini C, Cilotti A, Moretti M, Viacava P, et al. The

role of mean diffusivity (MD) as a predictive index of the response to chemotherapy in locally advanced breast cancer: a preliminary study. Eur Radiol 2010;20:303-8.

37. Negendank W. Studies of human tumors by MRS: a review. NMR Biomed 1992;5(5):303-24.

38. Bartella L, Morris EA, Dershaw DD, Liberman L, Thakur SB, Moskowitz C, et al. Proton MR spectroscopy with choline peak as malignancy marker improves positive predictive value for breast cancer diagnosis: preliminary study. Radiology 2006;239(3):686-92.

39. Baek HM, Chen JH, Nalcioglu O, Su MY. Proton MR spectroscopy for monitoring early treatment response of breast cancer to neo-adjuvant chemotherapy. Ann Oncol 2008;19(5): 1022-4.

40. Amin AL, Purdy AC, Mattingly JD, Kong AL, Termuhlen PM. Benign breast disease. Surg Clin North Am. 2013 Apr;93(2):299-308.

41. Guray M, Sahin AA. Benign breast diseases: classification, diagnosis, and management. Oncologist. 2006;11:435-49

42. Miltenburg DM, Speights Jr VO. Benign breast disease. Obstet Gynecol Clin North Am. 2008;35:285-300, ix.

43. Athanasiou, A., Aubert, E., Vincent Salomon, A., & Tardivon, A. (2014). Complex cystic breast masses in ultrasound examination. Diagnostic and Interventional Imaging, 95(2), 169-179.

44. Cho N, Moon WK, Chang JM, Kim SJ, Lyou CY, Choi HY: Aliasing artifact depicted on ultrasound (US)-elastography for breast cystic lesions mimicking solid masses. Acta Radiol. 2011;52:3-7.

45. Sakalecha, A. K., H Parameshwar, K. B., Savagave, S. G., & Naik, B. R. The Role of Ultrasonography and Elastography in Differentiating Benign From Malignant Breast Masses With Pathologic Correlation. Journal of Diagnostic Medical Sonography. 2022;38:226-234.

46. U C, Seror JY, Seror J. Management of a breast cystic syndrome: Guidelines. J Gynecol Obstet Biol Reprod. 2015 Dec;44(10):970-9.

47. Sabate J.M., Clotet M., Torrubia S.: Radiologic evaluation of breast disorders related to pregnancy and lactation. Radiographics. 2007; 27 (Suppl. 1): pp. S101- S124.

48. Sabate J.M., Clotet M., Torrubia S.: Radiologic evaluation of breast

disorders related to pregnancy and lactation. Radiographics. 2007; 27 (Suppl. 1): pp. S101- S124.

49. Cholot M, Dang-Tran KD, Castelain CS. Postpartum inflammatory breast tumour: necrotic lactating adenoma. Imagerie de la femme 2007;17:40-5.

50. Baker TP, Lenert JT, Parker J. Lactating adenoma: a diagnosis of exclusion. Breast J 2001;5:354-7.

51. Sumkin JH, Perrone AM, Harris KM. Lactating adenoma: US features and literature review. Radiology 1998;206:271-4.

52. Beyrouti MI, Boujelben S, Beyrouti R, Ben Amar M, Abid M, Louati D, et al. Pyog√©nic abc√©s of the breast: clinical and th√©peutic aspects. Gynecol Obstet Fertil. 2007 Jul-Aug;35(7-8):645-50.

53. Bretz-Grenier MF, Gros D, Bourjat P. Inflammatory breast outside the post partum period. Cours de perfectionnement post-universitaire. Journ√©es Fran√ßaises de Radiologie. Paris, 1997.

54. Khaled A, Saadi A, Jaziri M, Ben Romdhane K, Boussen H, Khattech R et al. La tuberculose mammaire: aspects radiocliniques √† proposde 70cas .Rev Im Med. 1992;4:755-758.

55. Delaloye JF, Brugger CR, Treboux AI, Anaye A, Meuwly JY. Abc√®s of the breast: privil√©gier la ponction aspiration √©choguid√©e. Rev Med Suisse. 2010 Oct 27;6(268):2010-2.

56. Boisserie-Lacroix M, Lafitte JJ, Sirben C, Latrabe V, Grelet P, Zeinoun R, Brun G. Inflammatory l√©sions of the breast. Contribution de l'√©chographie. J Chir 1993; 130 (10) : 408-415

57. Campassi C, Cilotti A, Moretti M, Bagnolesi P, De Liperi A, Bartolozzi C. High-frequency ultrasound (10-13 MHz) in inflammatory diseases of the breast. The Breast. 1996; 5: 351-357.

58. Karstrup S, Nolsoe C, Braband K, Nielsen KR et al. Ultrasonically guided percutaneous drainage of breast abscesses. Acta Radiol. 1990; 31: 157-159.

59. Marchant DJ. Inflammation of the breast. Obstet Gynecol Clin North Am. 2002;29:89-102.

60. Kamal RM, Hamed ST, Salem DS. Classification of inflammatory breast disorders and step by step diagnosis. Breast J. 2009;15(4):367-80.

61. Ayeva-Derman M, Perrotin F, Lefrancq T, et al. Idiopathic granulomatous mastitis. Review of the literature illustrated by 4 observations. J Gynecol Obstet

Biol Reprod. 1999;28(8):800-7.
62. Fletcher A, Magrath IM, Riddell RH, Talbot IC. Granulomatous mastitis: a report of seven cases. J Clin Pathol. 1982;35(9):941-5.
63. Kessler E, Wolloch Y. Granulomatous mastitis: a lesion clinically simulating carcinoma. Am J Clin Pathol. 1972;58(6):642-6.
64. Page DL, Anderson TJ. London: Churchill Livingston; 1987. Diagnostic histopathology of the breast; pp. 64-5.
65. Seo HR, Na KY, Yim HE, et al. Differential diagnosis in idiopathic granulomatous mastitis and tuberculous mastitis. J Breast Cancer. 2012; 15: 111-118
66. N. Raj N and others, Rheumatologists and breasts: immunosuppressive therapy for granulomatous mastitis, Rheumatology, Volume 43, Issue 8, August 2004, Pages 1055-1056.
67. DeHertogh DA, Rossof AH, Harris AA, Economou SG. Prednisone management of granulomatous mastitis. N Engl J Med. 1980 Oct 2;303(14):799-800.
68. Kim J, Tymms KE, Buckingham JM. Methotrexate in the management of granulomatous mastitis. ANZ J Surg. 2003 Apr;73(4):247-9.
69. Bogomoletz WV. Two cases of sclerosing lipogranuloma. Archives of Pathological Anatomy. 1975, Vol 23, Num 3, pp 249-51.
70. Denison CM, Ward VL, Lester SC, et al. Epidermal inclusion cysts of the breast: three lesions with calcifications. Radiology, 1997, vol. 204, no 2, p. 493-496.
71. Celik V, Unal E, Aydogan F, Sunamak O, Kusaslan R, Rasier R, et al. Epidermal inclusion cyst of the breast: clinical, radiologic, and pathologic correlation. BreastJ. 2004; 10:57.
72. Merajver SD, Sabel MS. Inflammatory breast cancer. In: Harris JR, Lippman ME, Morrow M, Osborne CK, editors. Diseases of the breast. Philadelphia: Lippincott Williams and Wilkins; 2004, p. 971-82.
73. Féger C, Leconte I, Fellah L. Imaging inflammatory cancers. Imagerie de la femme 2006;16:181-90.
74. Günhan-Bilgen I, Ûstün EE, Memis A. Inflammatory breast carcinoma: mammographic, ultrasonographic, clinical and pathological findings in 142 cases. Radiology 2002;223:829-38.
75. Yang WT, Le-Petross HT, Macapinlac H. Inflammatory breast cancer: PET/CT, MRI, mammography and sonography findings. Breast Cancer Res Treat 2008;109:417-26.

76. Lee KW, Chung SY, Kim HD. Inflammatory breast cancer: imaging findings. Clin Imaging 2005;29:22-5.

77. Stavros AT. Inflammatory carcinoma of the breast. In: Stavros AT, editor. Breast ultrasound. Philadelphia: LippincottWilliams andWilkins; 2004, p. 676-81.

78. Belli P, Costantini M, Romani M, Pastore G. Role of magnetic resonance imaging in inflammatory carcinoma of the breast. Rays 2002;27:299-305.

79. Rieber A, Tomczack RJ, Mergo PJ. MRI of the breast in the differential diagnosis of mastitis versus inflammatory carcinoma and follow-up. J Comput Assist Tomogr 1997;21:128-32.

80. Yasumura K, Ogawa K, Ishikawa H. Inflammatory carcinoma of the breast: characteristic findings of MR imaging. Breast Cancer 1997;4:161-9.

81. Chow CK. Imaging in inflammatory breast carcinoma. Breast Dis 2006;22:45-54.

82. Carbognin G, Calciolari C, Girardi V. Inflammatory breast cancer: MRimaging findings. Radiol Med 2010;115:70-82.

83. Le-Petross HT, Cristofanilli M, Carkaci S. MRI features of inflammatory breast cancer. AJR Am J Roentgenol 2011;197:769-76.

84. Féger C, Gilles R, Leconte I, Fellah L. Inflammatory breast imaging. EMC - Radiology and medical imaging - genitourinary - gynaeco-obstetrical - breast 2013;8(4):1-17 [Article 34-810-D-10].

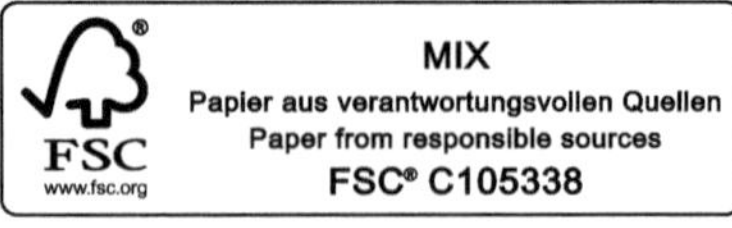

Printed by Books on Demand GmbH, Norderstedt / Germany